Contents

iii

Introduction to the Anatomy and Physiology of the Nervous System

DAVID BOWSHER

MA, MD, PhD

Reader in the Department of Anatomy,
University of Liverpool and Honorary Consultant,
Department of Medical and Surgical Neurology,
Walton Hospital, Liverpool

FOURTH EDITION

BLACKWELL SCIENTIFIC PUBLICATIONS
OXFORD LONDON EDINBURGH MELBOURNE

© 1967, 1970, 1975, 1979
Blackwell Scientific Publications
Editorial offices:
Osney Mead, Oxford, OX2 0EL
8 John Street, London, WC1N 2ES
9 Forrest Road, Edinburgh, EH1
  2QH
214 Berkeley Street, Carlton
Victoria 3053, Australia

First published 1967
Second edition 1970
Reprinted 1972
Third edition 1975
Fourth edition 1979
German edition 1973

Typeset by Enset Ltd
Midsomer Norton, Bath
printed in Great Britain at
Blackmore Press, Shaftesbury
and bound by
Kemp Hall Bindery, Oxford

DISTRIBUTORS

USA
  Blackwell Mosby Book
  Distributors
  11830 Westline Industrial Drive
  St Louis, Missouri 63141

Canada
  Blackwell Mosby Book
  Distributors
  86 Northline Road, Toronto
  Ontario, M4B 3E5

Australia
  Blackwell Scientific Book
  Distributors
  214 Berkeley Street, Carlton
  Victoria 3053

British Library
Cataloguing in Publication Data

Bowsher, David
  Introduction to the anatomy &
  physiology of the nervous system.
  —4th ed.
  1. Neurophysiology
  I. Title
  612'.8   QP355.2

  ISBN 0-632-00154-2

Preface to the Fourth Edition

For this edition, rather extensive changes have been made throughout the text, as well as to the format of the book. The chapter on blood supply has been completely re-written and illustrated with two new pictures. This chapter now presents a way of looking at the blood supply of the brain in a manner which differs entirely from the excellent topographical descriptions which are given in standard anatomy textbooks (at least one of which it is hoped that the student will read).

Alterations have also been made in a number of other chapters—though happily it has been possible to delete as well as to add. The principal new matter concerns axoplasmic transport, receptors with unmyelinated fibres, specific and non-specific sensory systems, skeletal motor systems, and neurosecretion in the hypothalamus. New illustrations and changes to old ones have been made by Mr. K. Biggs, to whom the author is dceply grateful Thanks are also due to Mr. F. W. Wallis, who prepared the index.

DAVID BOWSHER,

Liverpool 1979

Preface to First Edition

The forerunner of this small text first appeared in 1961, under the title of 'Introduction to Neuroanatomy'. In its original form, the book contained a fair amount of functional neuroanatomy, otherwise known as system neurophysiology. Many readers have however, asked for fuller treatment of the physiological aspects of the nervous system. This is the result. It includes most of the material from 'Introduction to Neuroanatomy', revised, where necessary, in the light of more recent knowledge; and, in addition, completely new matter on the physiology of the nervous system, which I hope has been successfully integrated with the contents of my original book. Chapters IV and V form an entirely new departure; I should like most sincerely to thank my friend and colleague Professor Denise Albe-Fessard, who provided the information on which these chapters are based, and most helpfully criticized their text. Coupled with my gratitude, I hasten to exonerate Professor Albe-Fessard from any culpability for error in their content, which must rest entirely on myself. My thanks are also due to Mr D. J. Kidd, who drew the illustrations which have been specially designed for this text. The pictures are deliberately diagrammatic or semi-diagrammatic, rather than being pictorial representations of what can be seen during actual dissection of the brain, or in stained sections of the central nervous system, as these are illustrated in several excellent atlases and larger textbooks.

Indeed, this book is not intended in any way to supplant larger textbooks, but to serve as an introduction to them. The author wishes to impress upon students, particularly those studying the nervous system for the first time, that the subject cannot be learned from this book alone; the text is meant to be used as an adjunct to lecture courses and brain dissection.

No references are given, because they clutter up the text, and students rarely want them; the author hereby apologizes to the many workers whose publications he has pirated without acknowledgment. A small select bibliography is given at the end; detailed references are to be found in all the larger textbooks, to which students should also refer for further data on any point requiring elaboration.

David Bowsher
Liverpool, 1967

CHAPTER ONE

Terminology

It would be idle to pretend that the study of the structure and function of the central nervous system (CNS) is not difficult. Perhaps one reason for this is that, compared with most other parts of the body, relatively little is known about the CNS. But the main reason is that the human CNS is the most highly developed and complicated in the whole animal kingdom. Our livers and our larynxes, for example, differ only very slightly from those of much more lowly beasts; but our brains are our crowning glory, and set us apart from and above the rest of brute creation. In studying our own brains, therefore, we have to try and begin to understand what it is that makes us 'only a little lower than the angels'. This is a difficult task, and a great challenge; but the effort is well repaid if it brings some comprehension of that which makes Man what he is.

Structure and function are more intricately bound up with one another in the CNS than in any other part of the body, and cannot be meaningfully separated from one another. Thus any book or course of lectures on the 'anatomy' of the CNS must of necessity deal to a large extent with its 'physiology'; and vice versa. The difference is only one of emphasis, and it would be well for students to realize at the outset that research workers in basic neurology are tackling essentially similar problems; they are only designated 'neuroanatomists' or 'neurophysiologists' according to the experimental methods that they use.

Most students, especially when approaching the CNS for the first time, find its gross morphology difficult to comprehend. There seem to be two main reasons for this. The first is that the nomenclature is confusing, containing many synonyms, and often meaningless; this latter because early observers were often unaware of the functional significance of what they observed, and so gave fanciful and functionally unhelpful names to what they saw. While many of the monstrous regiment of misnomers can now be discarded or replaced, many more of them are still left to plague the student of neurology in the second half of the twentieth century; the only thing he can do about this is to grin and bear it.

The second difficulty springs from the not unnatural attempt to visualize the morphology of the CNS in the same terms (or, as a neurologist might say, the same conceptual parameters) as the topographical anatomy of the rest of the body. Once the student realizes that he must take a completely different approach, the battle is already half won. For purposes of topographical anatomy, the vertical man is considered; then the directional signs superior, inferior, anterior and posterior are used. However, in the vertical man, the CNS is highly convoluted; so the first, and most important, thing to do is to dispense with these directional signs. Of course, the CNS has a true upper end, the forebrain, and a true lower end, the bottom of the spinal cord. When the CNS is considered along its length like this, it is called the **neuraxis**. By using the terms **rostral** (towards the beak) and **caudal** (towards the tail), direction up and down the neuraxis can be described irrespective of its bends and folds. It is important to realize that the directional signs are used only with reference to the neuraxis itself, and with no reference whatsoever to the rest of the body. The neuraxis has a front and a back, but the directions in which these face vary according to the bending and folding of the neuraxis; they are referred to, facultatively, as anterior or ventral, and posterior or dorsal; again, only with reference to the neuraxis itself, and not to the rest of the body. The neuraxis, like the rest of the body, has a midline, so the terms medial and lateral are employed in the usual way.

Sections cut at right angles to the long axis of the neuraxis are **coronal**. This again is irrespective of its bends, so that, for example, a coronal section of forebrain is at 90° from a coronal section of spinal cord; but they are both at right angles to the neuraxis. Similarly, sections parallel to the front and back of the neuraxis are **horizontal**; while vertical sections in the long axis of the CNS are called **sagittal** if in the midline, and **parasagittal** if lateral to the midline but parallel with the sagittal plane.

The most important directional and spatial terms are given in the preceding paragraphs. Most other terms will be defined as the text proceeds, but a few more may usefully be given at this juncture:

Ascending—running in a rostral direction.

Descending—running in a caudal direction.

Orthodromic—in the direction of a nerve fibre **away** from the parent cell body.

Antidromic—in the direction of a nerve fibre **towards** the parent cell body.

Nucleus—A collection of nerve cells having common connections and functions.

Afferent
- petal } —coming towards

Efferent
- fugal } —going away from

Kinaesthesia—the conscious sensation of joint movement.

Proprioception—nervous impulses set up by the lengthening or shortening of muscles.

Exteroceptive—coming from outside the body.

Enteroceptive—coming from inside the body.

Modality—Quality of stimulus.

CHAPTER TWO

Basic Cellular Elements and Development of the Nervous System

The nerve cell is specialized for impulse conduction and secretion, and it sacrifices many other biological functions to this end. It cannot reproduce itself, and its metabolism is so simple and immediate that it cannot live for more than a few minutes without oxygen. Its very high energy consumption is evidenced by the fact that mitochondria constitute nearly two thirds of the neurone's volume. It is probably the most delicate cell in the whole body, and requires a chemical environment even more constant than that of the plasma which bathes other cells.

As cells go, the nerve cell is fairly large (Fig. 1), though great variation is to be found in different parts of the central nervous

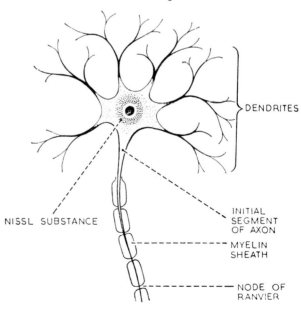

FIG. 1. Diagram of a nerve cell and its processes.

system (CNS). It contains a large nucleus, which has a nucleolus. The cytoplasm contains a granular substance which stains with basic (blue) dyes. Both the substance and the staining method are called after Nissl, who first described the phenomenon. The amount of **Nissl substance** (which in fact consists of ribosomes) in a cell diminishes after prolonged activity. Its regeneration appears to be dependent on the nucleolus. Attached to the cell body are a variable number of branching processes called **dendrites**. The area over which the dendrites of a single nerve cell extend is called the **dendritic field** of that cell.

In addition to the dendrites, each cell possesses a single process called the **axon** or nerve fibre. This may vary in length from less than a millimetre to over a yard. Any axon may or may not have one or more collateral branches whose destination may be quite different from that of the parent or stem axon (it may even turn back into the dendritic field of its own cell as a recurrent collateral).

The axon or collateral may remain with the CNS or pass out into a peripheral nerve. Those which end within the CNS do so by breaking up into a number of **terminal filaments** or **telo-dendria.** At the end of the telodendron is a small swelling called the **bouton terminal** or **synaptic knob.**

Neurones and their processes, up to and including axon terminals, contain microtubules (neurotubules) some 20–26 nm in diameter. Neurofilaments, 10 nm in diameter, are particularly evident in axons. Both types of structure may be concerned in the phenomenon of **axoplasmic transport**, whereby substances actively move along axons, both towards the terminals, and away from the terminals towards the cell body. Anterograde (somato-fugal) transport shows two peaks, at approximately 1 mm per day and 400 mm/day; the rapid transport includes substances such as proteins, while the slow bulk axonal flow includes substances with smaller molecules. Retrograde (somatopetal) transport has been chiefly studied with proteins, and seems to have a peak of activity at about 200 mm/day.

The bouton is classically in contact (contiguity not continuity) with the cell body or dendrite of another neurone, constituting an axosomatic or axodendritic **synapse** (Fig. 3).

The structure of the synaptic knob has also been elucidated by electron microscopy. The button is seen to contain a number of **synaptic vesicles** (Fig. 4). When a nervous impulse arrives at the button, it causes **transmitter substance** to be liberated from these vesicles; the details of its mode of action will be considered in Chapter 4.

The nerve cell and all its processes is called the **neurone**, and each neurone (of which the human nervous system contains some

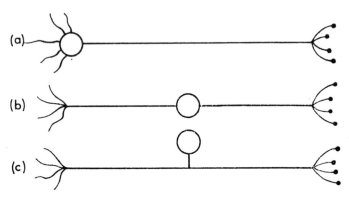

FIG. 2. Three common types of neurone (after Bodian and Hallowell Davis). In all cases, the dendritic ramifications, capable only of decremental electrotonic conduction, are at the left; the axonal portion is in the middle; and the telodendria and vesicle-containing synaptic knobs are at the right. Only the position of the cell body varies: (a) is the type most commonly found in the central nervous system; (b) is the bipolar type of neurone found in the retina and VIIIth cranial nerve; (c) is the pseudo-unipolar neurone characteristic of dorsal root and corresponding sensory cranial ganglia.

15–20 thousand million) is a self-contained and independent unit. Neurones whose cell bodies lie within the central nervous system are like that illustrated in Fig. 1, and have the cell body interposed between the dendrites and the axon. However, neurones whose cell bodies lie outside the CNS, and whose function is to conduct impulses from the periphery into the CNS, have the cell body as it were slid along the axon (Fig. 2), so that the dendrites run directly into the peripheral end of the axon; in nerves coming from the skin, the cell body (in the **dorsal root** or corresponding **sensory cranial nerve ganglion**) is on a side branch of the axon.

The neurone doctrine teaches that nervous conduction, under normal conditions, starts at the dendritic end of the axon (whether this be the cell body or not) and travels towards the telodendria with their terminal buttons. Thus it will be seen that the function of the cell body, apart from providing a large area of membrane surface (see Chapter 4) is chiefly to ensure the maintenance of the various processes and their branches, which constitute the essential conducting mechanism of the neurone. The conditions under which the nervous impulse is generated and conducted, as well as the way in which impulses cross the synaptic junction between neurones, will be dealt with in chapter 4.

Two types of neurones within the CNS should be considered. First is the primitive **isodendritic** neurone (Fig. 3) with long straight dendrites. Its axon bears many collateral branches which go off in different directions to establish small numbers of synaptic contacts with large numbers of secondary neurones.

Since the number of synaptic knobs in contact with a neurone of any type is very large (up to 50,000 in some instances), it is usually the case that the more or less synchronous activation of a large number of synapses is necessary to fire the neurone; impulses arriving at one, or a very small number of synapses, will usually be ineffective.

Such neurones are generally found in the primitive reticular core of the neuraxis, forming the non-specific or extralemniscal system (see Chapter 11) and hypothalamus (Chapter 15). The pattern of their widely distributed efferents and heterogeneous afferents makes it evident that impulses arriving from a single afferent source are unlikely to fire a secondary neurone; but that each neurone is open to a very large number of afferent inputs, and able through its widely divergent output to influence the activity of large numbers of secondary neurones.

Second is the **tufted** neurone (Fig. 3) with a smaller but denser bushy dendritic field. Its axon has a small number of collateral branches which tend to make multiple, concentrated, synaptic contacts with small numbers of secondary neurones. It is found

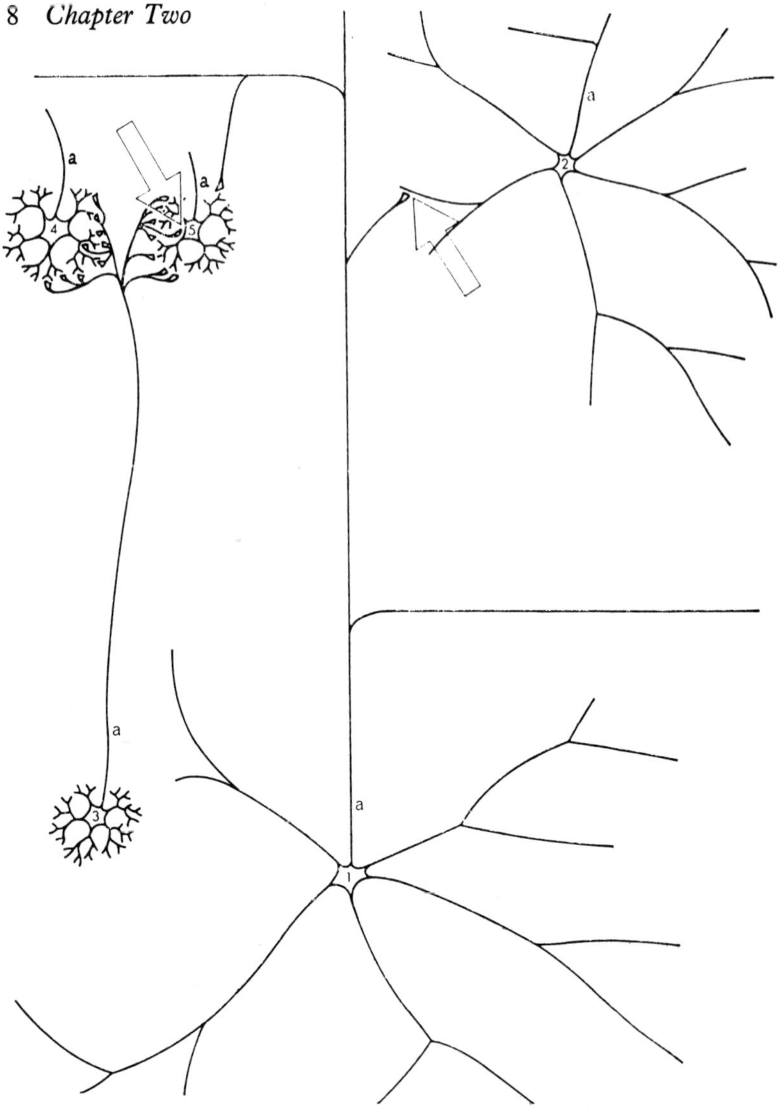

FIG. 3. 1 and 2 are isodendritic neurones, whose axons (a) have many collateral branches, giving a small number of contacts to a large number of secondary neurones, including those of the tufted type (3, 4 and 5). The axons (a) of the latter establish a large number of contacts with a small number of secondary neurones of their own type. The right-hand arrow indicates an axodendritic synapse, while the left-hand arrow is pointing to an axosomatic synapse.

in the recently evolved nuclei belonging to the specific or lemniscal systems (Chapter 10). The nature of the concentrated afferents and efferents means that such cells influence only a relatively small number of secondary neurones, but do so in a manner which is fairly certain to cause the latter to fire; this is the morphological basis of so-called **synaptic security.**

Within certain specific relay centres of the brain, such as the thalamus (Chapters 8 and 12) a type of **interneurone** is found which sometimes does not even possess an axon. Some of its processes, however, contain synaptic vesicles and enter into the composition of a **synaptic glomerulus** where they are post-synaptic to some structures and pre-synaptic to others (Fig. 4). All known interneurones of this type are inhibitory, and their vesicle-containing processes are probably responsible for the phenomenon known as **pre-synaptic inhibition** (see p. 32 below).

Every axon and its branches, as far as the terminal filament, is covered with a layer of white fatty substance known as **myelin,** except the first little bit, where it arises from the axon hillock; this is known as the **initial segment.** The larger the axon the thicker its myelin sheath—the largest nerve fibres in the human CNS are about 20 μm in diameter (including the axon sheath). Roughly speaking, large axons arise from large nerve cells and vice versa. The smallest axons (from 0.5 to 1.0 μm in diameter, including sheath) have only a very thin film of myelin, which could not be seen with the fat stains formerly used for myelin, and so these, to this day, are called 'unmyelinated axons'. The larger axons, both inside and outside the central nervous system, have their myelin arranged like a string of sausages, separated by the **nodes of Ranvier.** If the myelin is not developed (and in some cases it is not laid down until after birth) or destroyed (as in some diseases), the axon will not conduct nervous impulses. Although this sounds very like an insulator, it should be remembered that nervous conduction differs from electrical in several important respects. It will be sufficient here to state that the speed of conduction in any axon is proportional to its diameter, the largest axons conducting most rapidly (about 120 metres/sec or 270 m.p.h.) and the smallest

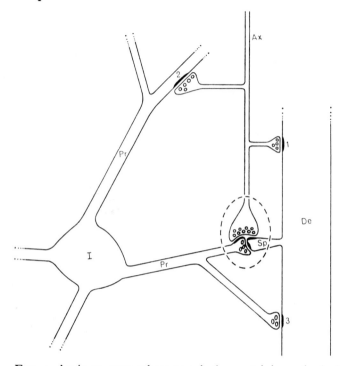

FIG. 4. Ax is an axon whose terminals, containing spherical vesicles, make excitory synapses with the dendrite (De) of a relay neurone at 1 and with a process (Pr) of an inhibitory interneurone (I) at 2; this process in its turn has endings containing ovoid vesicles, one of which makes an inhibitory synapse with the dendrite at 3. The region within the dashed outline is a synaptic glomerulus, partly or wholly encapsulated by glial processes (not shown). In the glomerulus, an axon terminal is presynaptic to both a spine (Sp) of the relay neurone dendrite and to a terminal of an interneurone process, while the latter is also presynaptic to the dendritic spine.

most slowly (about 0.5 metre/sec or 1 m.p.h.); but that the speed of conduction in even the largest axon is some three million times slower than the rate of flow of electricity. When a **nervous** impulse is generated in a nerve cell, the first **electrical** change is observed in the initial segment of the axon. Further morphological information about axons will be given in Chapter 4, when the physiological correlates are explained.

Axons outside the central nervous system have a further covering outside the myelin, known as the **neurilemma** or sheath of Schwann. Their telodendria end in synaptic contact with an **effector** organ—usually a muscle, but sometimes a gland; in the case of striated muscle, the termination is known as a **motor end plate.**

If a nerve cell body is destroyed (e.g. by anoxia, by toxins, or by virus infection such as poliomyelitis) the whole neurone dies. If the axon is cut, the neurone dies unless its continuity is re-established. In the case of peripheral axons, new axon filaments will grow along the neurilemmal sheath from the central end of the neurone and so repair will be effected. But in the CNS, where there is no neurilemmal sheath, repair is so exceptional that for practical purposes it may be discounted.

Three types of supporting cell are developed from the neuroectoderm which gives rise to the neurone. The first of these is the **ependymal cell,** which lines the central canal and ventricles of the neuraxis (brain and spinal cord). It has a long peripheral process which may reach out to the external aspect of the neuraxis.

The two other types of cell developed from neuroectoderm make up the most of the **neuroglia** (but which also includes microglia, vide infra). It should be noted immediately that within the CNS, neuroglia outnumber neurones in the ratio of about 10:1.

Scattered throughout the CNS, but particularly among the nerve cells (grey matter), are the **astrocytes.** These cells have a number of processes, some of which may be in contact with neurones, and at least one of which is in contact with the wall of a capillary blood vessel. It is thought that these cells may be concerned with the transport of metabolites in both directions between the neurones and the blood stream.

Rather smaller cells, with fewer processes, known as **oligodendrocytes,** have a tendency to lie in rows between the axis cylinders (myelin sheaths) of nerve fibres. It is now known that the myelin sheaths of axons within the CNS consist of oligodendroglial processes wrapped round the axons in a helical fashion, like a Swiss roll. In fact, the node of Ranvier represents the interruption between the processes of two separate oligodendroglial elements.

The whole neuraxis is richly permeated with blood vessels—one fifth of the total output of the heart is normally taken up by the CNS. Those wandering macrophages which normally pass in and out of capillaries to perform their scavenging functions take on a peculiar morphology in the CNS, where they are known as **microglia**. Their characteristic appearance in the CNS, so different from their appearance elsewhere, may be due to the peculiar chemical environment to which they are subjected in the CNS.

The millions of neurones which make up the CNS tend to be grouped in certain predetermined ways, and in studying their arrangement, we pass from the microscopical to the gross anatomy of the neuraxis. At the simplest level the nerve cells tend to be congregated in a central core, while longitudinally running axons lie outside them. This arrangement is still to be found in the spinal cord, although the cells appear to be in a butterfly shape on cross-section, rather than a circle. Owing to the glistening white appearance of the myelin in the fresh state, the bundles of nerve fibres are known as **white matter**. The collections of nerve cells, cn the other hand, have a reddish-brown appearance, and so are l n)wn as **grey matter** (Figs. 5a and 5b).

As the grey and white matter are followed rostrally into the brain, the arrangement becomes rather more complicated. This is mainly due to the fact that the bundles of white fibres, instead of all running longitudinally, now begin, in part, to run transversely in all directions across the brain stem, and so cut up the grey matter into a series of more or less discrete and apparently disconnected lumps. The forebrain (cerebral hemispheres) and cerebellum show an additional feature, which is the development of an extra layer of grey matter on their external surfaces; this is known as **cortex** (Fig. 5c).

The whole CNS is developed from embryonic **neuroectoderm**. In the primitive **neural tube**, the grey matter is segregated into a dorsal **alar lamina**, and a ventral **basal lamina**. The cells of the alar lamina are sensory in function—that is, they are concerned with the reception and or transmission of impulses arriving from outside the CNS, while the cells of the basal lamina are **motor**—their axons pass outside the CNS and supply muscular or glandular

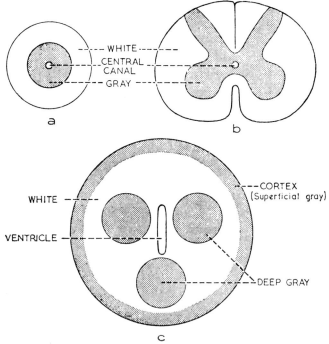

FIG. 5. Diagrams to show the relationship of grey (shaded) to white matter in (a) the primitive neural tube, (b) the definitive spinal cord, and (c) the cerebellum and cerebral hemispheres.

tissue. In the mature CNS, the cells of the alar and basal laminae form discontinuous columns running the whole length of the neuraxis. Primitively, these cell columns have a strict dorso-ventral arrangement within each lamina and this arrangement persists in the mature spinal cord. The cell columns with their adult derivatives, from dorsal to ventral, are listed on p. 14. This list may usefully be referred to when reading the later chapters of the book.

The brain stem—medulla oblongata, pons, midbrain, and diencephalon—undergoes various flexures, and internal rearrangements of the cell columns, but it contains elements from both laminae. But the cerebral hemispheres (forebrain, telencephalon) and the cerebellum develop from alar lamina only. In both these parts of the CNS, the cortex should be regarded as an added luxury, having no strictly developmental continuity with either lamina.

	Cell column	Spinal cord representative	Brain stem representative	Fibres in cranial nerves	Structures innervated	
ALAR LAMINA	1. Special afferent	Nil	Cochlear nuclei Vestibular nuclei (Rostral) solitary nucleus	(I, II) VIII VII, IX, X	Special sense organs	S E N S O R Y
	2. Somatic afferent	Dorsal horn cells	Principal sensory and spinal (descending) Trigeminal nuclei	V	Skin and deep somatic structures	
	3. Visceral afferent	? Intermedio-lateral horn T1-L2, S2, 3, 4	(Caudal) solitary nucleus	V IX, X	Viscera	
BASAL LAMINA	4. Visceral efferent	Intermedio-lateral horn T1-L2, S2, 3, 4	Edinger-Westphal nucleus of III Dorsal nucleus of vagus	III VII, IX, X	Smooth and cardiac muscle; glands	M O T O R
	5. Branchiomotor	(Spinal accessory nucleus)	Trigeminal and facial motor nuclei Nucleus ambiguus	V, VII IX, X, XI	Striated muscle derived from branchial arch mesoderm	
	6. Somatic efferent	Ventral horn cells	Oculomotor, trochlear, abducent and hypoglossal nuclei	III, IV VI, XII	Striated muscle derived from myotomes	

CHAPTER THREE

Membranes and Spaces:
Blood and Cerebrospinal Fluid

Just as the abdominal and thoracic viscera are invaginated into double-layered serous membranes (peritoneum and pleura), so is the neuraxis. The lower end of the spinal cord (opposite the second lumbar vertebra) is tethered to the back of the coccyx by a strand of primitive neuroectoderm, the **filum terminale** (Fig. 6). It is through this caudal end that the neuraxis is invaginated into its membranes, which are called the **leptomeninges.** The visceral layer is closely adherent to the nervous substance, and forms the adventitial coat of its blood vessels; it is called the **pia mater.** Around the middle part of the filum terminale (opposite the second piece of the sacrum) the pia mater becomes continuous with the parietal layer, which is called the **arachnoid mater.** Between the arachnoid and the pia maters is the **subarachnoid space** which contains **cerebrospinal fluid**; it is crossed by some strands of leptomeninx called **arachnoid trabeculations.** The portion of the subarachnoid space which lies caudal to the lower end of the spinal cord (Fig. 6) is known as the **lumbar sac** or **theca**; it is from here that cerebrospinal fluid is withdrawn for sampling by **lumbar puncture.**

Covering the outer surface of the arachnoid mater is a fibrous membrane called the **dura mater** or **pachymeninx.** This bears the same relationship to the arachnoid as does the fibrous capsule of a joint to the outer or parietal layer of the synovial membrane.

The whole neuraxis and its membranes are covered by bone, the spinal cord lying within the vertebral canal of the vertebral column and the brain in the cranial cavity of the skull. Because of their arrangement in two tables separated by diploë, the bones of the cranial vault have a periosteal membrane on both their inner and outer surfaces. The periosteum (endosteum) of the inner table is adherent to the cranial dura mater, except at points where the two are separated by venous sinuses. For this reason the cranial endosteum has confusingly and unfortunately come to be called the 'outer layer of the dura mater', while the true dura, which is of course continuous through the foramen magnum with the spinal dura, is in this situation called the 'inner layer of the

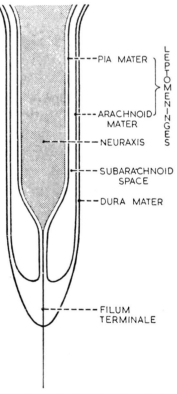

FIG. 6. Diagram to show the invagination of the neuraxis from its caudal end (spinal cord) into its serous membranes (leptomeninges). The lumbar theca constitutes the portion of the subarachnoid space below the spinal cord.

cranial dura'. The important point to grasp is that blood vessels which are said to lie **between** the layers of the cranial dura (intradural) are in the same morphological plane as those which lie **outside** the spinal dura (extradural) (Fig. 7).

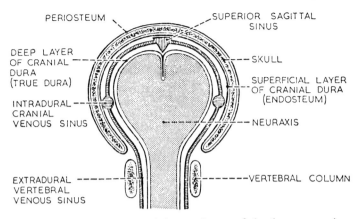

FIG. 7. The relationship of the two layers of the dura mater in the cranial cavity. Note the continuity of the inner layer (true dura) with the spinal dura.

Running the length of the spinal cord is the ependyma-lined **central canal**. In the lower brain stem this dilates into a cavity, the **fourth ventricle** (Fig. 8) of which the floor is formed by the lower brain stem and the roof by the cerebellum. At its rostral end, surrounded by the midbrain, this ventricle narrows off again into a canal called the **cerebral aqueduct**, which opens rostrally into another cavity, the **third ventricle**, which is the cavity of the most rostral part of the brain stem (diencephalon). The forebrain or cerebral hemispheres lie lateral rather than rostral to this part of the brain stem; each hemisphere contains a cavity, the **lateral ventricle**, which communicates medially with the third ventricle. This whole canalicular and ventricular system communicates through three holes in the fourth ventricle (one median in the roof, and two lateral) with the subarachnoid space. Thus the spaces inside and outside the neuraxis are continuous with one another, and all contain cerebrospinal fluid (CSF). This fluid is of very constant composition, which differs in several important respects from that of plasma (or even of a plasma filtrate). It certainly acts as a fluid buffer for the neuraxis, and probably has important metabolic functions as well.

The blood vessels of the subarachnoid space are invested with pia mater, which forms their adventitial coat. Many of the smaller

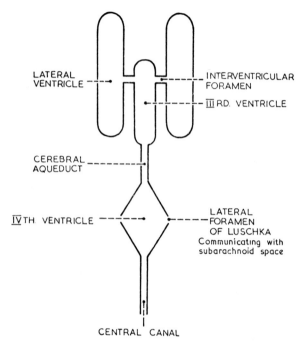

FIG. 8. Diagram of the ependyma-lined ventricular and canalicular system of the neuraxis. The only communications with the subarachnoid space are in the fourth ventricle.

vessels (venules) have an incomplete tunica media, so that vascular endothelium and pia are in direct contact. As the vessels on the surface of the neuraxis enter into its depths, they carry their pial sheath with them. In the case of the larger vessels, this sheath may at first be separable from the vessel wall, thus allowing the subarachnoid space to be prolonged as a **perivascular space**, which is finally obliterated by blending of the pia with the vascular wall. Thus there is absolutely no connection between the subarachnoid space and a real or imaginary perineuronal space (Fig. 9).

In the case of the arteries which enter the cerebral ventricles, there is a modification of this pattern. The arterioles are thrown into a highly convoluted plexus, while the ependyma covering them becomes modified so that its cells form a cubical or columnar type of glandular epithelium. The whole complex is known as a

choroid plexus and is concerned with the active secretion of at least some of the constituents of CSF.

If certain dyes (e.g. trypan blue) be injected into the systemic blood stream, all the tissues of the body with the exception of the CNS become stained with the dye. Because of this failure of the dye to penetrate the CNS or CSF, the existence of a blood-brain barrier has been postulated. This obstacle to free diffusion is now believed to be due to the high packing density of cellular elements within the CNS, so that, under normal conditions, there is very little extracellular or intercellular space into which large molecules from the blood could diffuse. The barrier, consisting of apposed

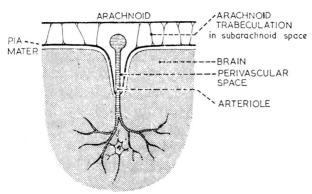

FIG. 9. The relationship of the subarachnoid and perivascular spaces.

cell membranes, is selective, in that it allows some substances, e.g. water, to pass freely.

CSF appears to have a dual origin. Some constituents are actively secreted by the choroid plexus, others pass into the sub-arachnoid space or ventricular system by simple diffusion across the limiting membranes.

There is some evidence that sodium, for example, is secreted by the choroid plexus in hypertonic solution; therefore the entry of water by diffusion should be regarded as essentially an osmotic process, designed to re-establish the isotonicity of CSF as a whole. The fluid is largely absorbed into the veins of the pia and sub-arachnoid space (lepto-meningo-vascular absorption), but some escapes into the lymphatic system by passing along the meningeal sheaths of cranial and spinal nerves (perineuro-lymphatic absorption). It should be noted that there are no lymphatics in the CNS itself.

The veins of the brain and cranial subarachnoid space end by piercing the dura mater to flow into the venous sinuses which lie between the true dura and the cranial endosteum (intradural venous sinuses). At the points where these veins pierce the dura, a little knot of arachnoid is frequently carried through the dura into the venous sinus; these **arachnoid villi** or **granulations**, which increase in size with age, are mostly found in the superior sagittal and transverse sinuses. They were formerly thought to be a special mechanism for the absorption of CSF, but it is probable that this is not in fact their principal function, although some CSF undoubtedly passes through them into the venous sinuses. The cranial venous sinuses eventually drain into the internal jugular vein and thence into superior vena cava.

The veins of the spinal cord and spinal subarachnoid space form plexuses around the emergent nerve roots, which join large thin-walled venous sinuses which lie outside the dura in the vertebral canal. These sinuses are connected with the cranial venous sinuses, which lie in the same morphological plane, but their main drainage is through the intervertebral foramina into the ascending lumbar and posterior intercostal veins. These eventually join the azygos system, so that virtually all the blood from the whole neuraxis eventually drains into the superior vena cava. This means that pressure changes in the craniovertebral subarachnoid space, reflected back from rhythmic changes in intrathoracic pressure, are in the same phase throughout the system. If this were not so (i.e. if the cranial and vertebral spaces reflected superior and inferior caval, intrathoracic and intra-abdominal pressure changes respectively), cerebrospinal fluid would whoosh up and down the subarachnoid space like water slapping against the sides of a boat.

CHAPTER FOUR

Generation, Conduction, and Transmission of the Nervous Impulse

An excitable tissue is composed of cells which respond to an external **stimulus** in a manner specific to the type of tissue—in the case of the **neurone, emission of an impulse**, of **muscle, contraction**, and of **gland, secretion**. The effective stimulus may be artificial or natural. Artificial stimuli include a number of chemical and physical agents; the most frequently used for experimental purposes is the application of electric current, but some excitable tissues, such as certain mammalian smooth muscles, and the electric organs of marine fish, are electrically inexcitable. The **response**, in the case of nerve and muscle, is of an explosive nature, and depends on the bioelectric characteristics of the cell membrane. The cell membranes of neurones and muscle fibres are double-layered structures between 15 and 25 nm thick (the space between the layers being 6–7 nm).

The **Resting Membrane** is semipermeable. Large particles like organic molecules cannot pass across it; on the other hand it allows the passage of small ions. The protoplasm inside the membrane performs metabolic work in order to retain potassium (K^+) ions inside the cell and extrudes sodium (Na^+) ions to the exterior. This is brought about by the coupled sodium and potassium pumps, which are a general physiological phenomenon, being found for example also in red blood corpuscles and kidney tubule cells.

In addition to these pumping mechanisms, the actual permeability of the membrane to these ions must be considered. This depends upon the electrical charge on the membrane. The potential difference which must be applied to the membrane in order to render it impermeable to each ion is known as the **equilibrium potential** for that ion. In the case of the membrane of the cat spinal motoneurone the relevant equilibrium potentials are:

Na^+	$-60mV$	(the direction of the
K^+	$+90mV$	sign being relative to
Cl^-	$+70mV$	the inside of the cell)

Now if the actual potential difference across the cell membrane (i.e. between the inside and the outside of the cell) be measured, it is found generally to lie between $+40$ and $+100$ mV. This is known as the **resting** or **membrane potential***; in the case of the cat motoneurone cited above it is in fact $+70$ mV. Hence it is 20 mV below the equilibrium potential for K^+ and 130mV $(-60+70)$ above that for Na^+. These differences represent, in electrical terms, the amount of work which must be done by the sodium and potassium pumps to maintain the differences of concentration of Na^+ and K^+ ions on either side of the cell membrane. For example, actual concentrations, in millimoles, inside and outside the cat motoneurone are:

	External	*Internal*
Na^+	150	15
K^+	5·5	150
Cl^-	125	9

It will be seen that there is a reasonable balance in the concentration of internal and external cations (Na^+ and K^+), while there seems to be a huge disequilibrium of anions (Cl^-). This is in fact balanced by the presence inside the membrane of organic (protein) anions.

The resting membrane is much more permeable to K^+ than to Na^+; but the rate of diffusion of these two ions in opposite directions is almost equal, because the electromotive force acting on Na^+ ions (130 mV) is so much greater than that acting on K^+ ions (20 mV).

These electrochemical forces maintain the resting membrane in a polarized state, so that it is like a battery with its positive pole

---

* Note—all the phenomena known in neurophysiology as **potentials** are in reality potential **differences**.

(anode) on its outer surface and negative pole (cathode) on the inner surface (Fig. 10). So long as the membrane is intact, the circuit is open and no current flows between the poles. However, if the properties of the membrane are changed at some point, so that a reduced resistance appears, a flow of current will be established, such that negative charges pass to the outside and positive charges to the inside. The movement of charged ions across the interrupted membrane reduces the potential difference between the two surfaces at this point; the membrane is said to become **depolarized**.

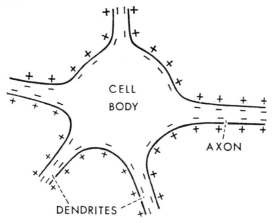

FIG. 10. A nerve cell body with the proximal portions of its axon and dendrites, showing the charges on the membrane in the resting state.

This local depolarization can be brought about by mechanical destruction of the membrane, in which case it is of course permanent. It can also be caused to occur reversibly in most, though not all, excitable tissues by the passage of an electrical current between a pair of **stimulating electrodes** applied to the outer surface of the membrane; this current must be sufficiently strong to penetrate the membrane in its passage from anode to cathode. If it does this, the membrane under the cathode becomes depolarized by the outflowing current.

However, in the case of naturally-occurring stimulation taking place at a point of contact between two excitable elements, the increase in membrane permeability (and hence depolarization) seems to be brought about by the action of a chemical substance which is secreted onto the membrane at a particular point of contact between two excitable elements. In neuro-neuronal contacts this is the **synapse**, and in contacts between nerve fibres and striated muscle it is the **motor end-plate**. At the motor end-plate, the **transmitter substance** secreted by the nerve terminal is known to be acetylcholine (ACh); it is also believed to be the active substance concerned in at least some synapses At junctions between sympathetic autonomic nerves and smooth muscle, on the other hand, the transmitter substance is usually nor-adrenaline

The membrane upon which the transmitter substance acts at the neuro-muscular junction is the membrane of the muscle fibre

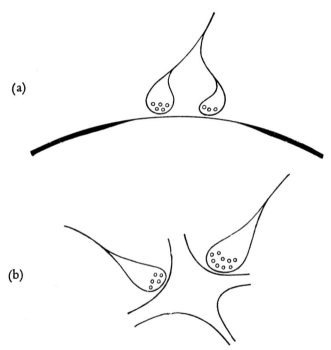

(a)

(b)

FIG. 11. Boutons terminaux, containing synaptic vesicles, in near-contact with the post-synaptic membrane of a striated muscle cell (a) and a nerve cell body (b).

(Fig. 11*a*) (sarcolemma); at the neuro-neuronal contact it is the post-synaptic membrane (Fig. 11*b*). In either case, the partially depolarized region of muscle or neurone membrane is negative with respect to the outer surface of the intact portion of the membrane. A potential difference is therefore set up between the two parts of the membrane. This is known, in the case of the neuro-neuronal contact, as the **post-synaptic potential,** and in the case of the neuromuscular junction as the **end-plate potential**. It must be emphasized that these potentials are (i) **local**, and (ii) **graduable**.

Because of the continuity of the membrane, this change in potential spreads from the point at which it is set up; this decre-

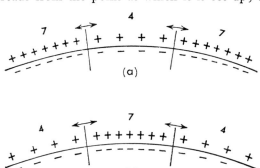

FIG. 12. A portion of neuronal membrane, divided into three equal parts. In (a), the central part is depolarized with respect to the adjacent regions, while in (b) it is hyperpolarized.

mental spread, called **electrotonus**, is variable, depending on the extent to which the membrane potential is changed at the point of maximal effect (i.e., depolarized—or, in the case of inhibition, hyperpolarized (Fig. 12)). The distance along which electrotonus spreads in the membrane is related not only to its initial size, but also to the capacitance properties of the membrane.

If the local change of potential provoked by natural or electrical stimulation or synaptic transmission is powerful enough, it leads to the appearance of an **action potential,** which is propagated along a neurone (causing a nervous message to be carried) (Fig. 13), or along a muscle fibre (causing it to contract). In a neurone with

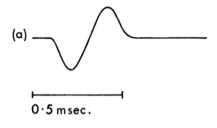

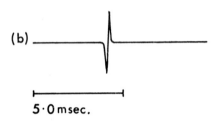

FIG. 13. Electrical recording of an action potential (spike), taken on different time bases; (b) is ten times faster than (a).

a resting potential of 70 mV, an action potential usually develops when the membrane potential has been lowered (depolarized) to about 55–60 mV. Once this critical point is reached, the production of a self-propagating action potential becomes inevitable. The increase in the permeability of the membrane makes it behave as though it had been transitorily breached. Na^+ ions from the external medium which come avalanching in not only annul the resting potential difference normally existing across the membrane, but actually reverse it, so that the inside of the neurone or muscle fibre at this point becomes positive with respect to the outside (Fig. 14). Because of the concentration gradient, K^+ ions equally pass out to the exterior. These events occur too rapidly for the relatively slow sodium-potassium pump mechanisms to keep up with them.

In this situation of reversed polarity, a current flow will immediately be set up between this depolarized region and adjoining regions of normal polarity (Fig. 14). This **local circuit** will flow out through the normal part of the membrane which thus becomes a source, and becomes depolarized and hence permeable to a sufficient extent for the ion-exchange phenomenon to re-occur. But by the same token, the local current will be returning through the originally depolarized part of the membrane, so tending to repolarize it; indeed, there is a temporary overswing, so that for a short time this part of the membrane becomes slightly hyperpolarized (in the direction of the equilibrium potential for K^+).

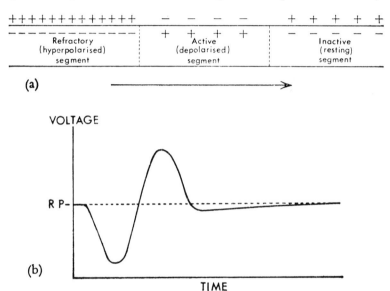

(a)

(b)

FIG. 14(a). Diagram of nervous conduction in an unmyelinated axon, spread out in space. (b) The same action potential recorded at a single point on the axon, and therefore spread out in time. R.P. = Resting potential.

The newly depolarized region sets up a local current with the next segment of the nerve or muscle fibre, and so the process travels on in a self-propagating fashion.

In this way, local depolarizing circuits may propagate an action potential along a nerve or muscle fibre. In the case of so-called unmyelinated nerve fibres (which in fact are covered with a very thin layer of myelin, some 8 nm thick), the action potential travels at a velocity of from 0·7 to 2·0 metres/sec., and in mammalian striated muscle fibres about 5·0 metres/sec. It can be shown that the rate of propagation in unmyelinated nerve fibre is proportional to the square root of the diameter of the fibre—so that for a four-fold increase in diameter, for example, the conduction velocity is only doubled.

In myelinated nerve fibres, because of the high resistance of myelin, the nerve fibre can be regarded as being sealed off on its outer surface, except as the nodes of Ranvier, so that electro-chemical ionic movements are confined to the nodes. Thus the local currents are set up between nodes, and the depolarizing process jumps from node to node; this is known as **saltatory conduction** (Fig. 15). In myelinated fibres the velocity of con-duction is directly proportional to the diameter of the fibre, and is also dependent on the distance between the nodes; in the peri-pheral nerves, this distance is about 1 mm in the small myelinated fibres, 2 or 3 mm in the larger ones. It can be calculated that con-duction velocity in small (Aδ) myelinated fibres, in metres per second, is 4·5 times the diameter in μm, while in large (Aα, Aβ; Groups I and II) fibres it is 5·7 times the diameter. The efficacy of saltatory conduction is shown by the fact that a myelinated fibre of 2 μm diameter conducts five or six times more rapidly than an unmyelinated axon of the same thickness.

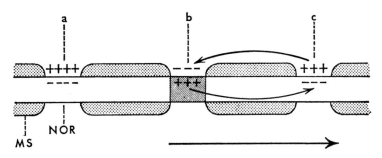

FIG. 15. Saltatory conduction in a myelinated axon. MS: myelin sheath; NOR: Node of Ranvier. At node (b) the membrane is active (depolarized); at (c) it is resting (inactive), while at (a) it is hyperpolarized (refractory). Cf. Fig. 14a, where the activity is passing along the whole length of the membrane, instead of jumping from node to node.

If the action potential is recorded from a fixed point on the nerve or muscle fibre, it will have a certain duration in time. For myelinated nerve fibres, this is usually about 0·5 ms; for unmyelinated nerve and striated muscle fibres, about 2·0 ms. Another way of stating this is to say that, at any given moment, the activity must occupy a given length of fibre—which may be as much as 6 cm in the largest mammalian nerve fibres, though only a few millimetres in the smallest.

When the wave of depolarization causing transitory membrane permeability has passed, metabolic processes restore the normal resting state ion concentrations on the two sides of the membrane. It is important to realize that only a tiny portion of the total ion content of the fibre is involved in the electrochemical activity of the action potential; it has been calculated that only one millionth of the K^+ ions in an axon pass out of the fibre during the passage of a single action potential. During the process of electro-chemical re-formation (recovery) of the membrane, it is inexcitable, and is thus said to be **refractory**.

If an artificial depolarizing current sufficiently large to cause the appearance of a propagated action potential be applied to a point somewhere in the middle of a long axon, the action potential will travel in both directions—out towards the axon terminals (**orthodromic conduction**) and inwards towards the cell body and dendrites (**antidromic conduction**). What determines the direction of propagation under physiological conditions is merely the point at which depolarization is brought about; and this (in the case of neurones) is on the cell body (by axo-somatic synapses) or dendrites (by axo-dendritic synapses). Thus natural conduction along an axon is always towards the terminal buttons (i.e. orthodromic). The arrival of the impulse at the axon terminal causes it to liberate transmitter substance. If the transmitter substance be excitatory (E-substance), it brings about a certain degree of depolarization in the post-synaptic membrane (post-synaptic and end-plate potentials).

In the case of the neuromuscular junctions in striated muscle, a single impulse travelling along an axon supplying a number of muscle fibres (motor unit) causes the liberation of enough ACh to bring about sufficient depolarization for a muscular potential to be generated, and therefore for the muscle fibres to contract.

This is a very simple case. It may sometimes occur at neuro-neuronal contacts in the central nervous system. But often several presynaptic impulses are required in order to set up sufficient post-synaptic depolarization for an action potential to be generated. In this case, each of these impulses is said to be **sub-liminal** (below threshold). But as the post-synaptic potential has a certain duration in time, the arrival of a further subliminal impulse or impulses within this time will have an additive effect, so that the critical threshold of post-synaptic depolarization is reached, and firing occurs (i.e. an action potential is generated). This is known as **temporal summation**.

Temporal summation could happen if a series of impulses arrived in succession at the same synapse. Another manner in which a series of subliminal stimuli can cause firing depends upon the fact that the depolarization of the post-synaptic potential spreads along the membrane beyond the point of actual synaptic contact. Thus the simultaneous arrival of a number of subliminal impulses, each one arriving in a different axon terminal, may bring about sufficient depolarization to cause firing; this is **spatial summation**. The morphological basis for this can be seen in the fact that the cat motoneurone, for example, is known to have some 1500 axon terminals in contact with its cell body (soma) and proximal dendrites; there is thus **convergence** of a number of axons on to a single post-synaptic membrane.

In all the cases described above, it is implicit that the transmitter substance brings about depolarization, and is excitatory (E-substance). At some neuro-neuronal junctions, the E-substance is ACh; but this is not so in all cases, so it is preferable to refer to E-substance than to a specific chemical when considering the phenomenon of excitation in general. When considering the passage of a nervous message along a chain of neurones, account must be taken not only of the **conduction time** taken by the passage of an impulse along a single neurone, but also of the time necessary for the liberation of transmitter substance and the time necessary for it to depolarize the post-synaptic membrane sufficiently to fire off an action potential. This time is known as **synaptic delay**, and in mammals is minimally of the order of o·5–o·7 ms. It should be noted that chemical mediation across the synaptic gap results in a considerable energy boost, in comparison to the electrical energy of the conducted impulse in the axon. Thus chemical transmission is more efficient than purely electrical synaptic transmission, such as occurs between some invertebrate neurones.

Liberated transmitter substance is normally very rapidly destroyed *in situ* by the action of enzymes (cholinesterase in the case of ACh). At the time when the axon membrane is completely depolarized, during the generation or passage of action potential it obviously cannot be depolarized any further, and so it is inexcitable; this is known as the **absolute refractory period**. Following the absolute refractory period, while the membrane is undergoing physiological restoration to electrochemical equilibrium, there occurs the **relative refractory period**, during which a supraliminal stimulus would be required to set off an action potential; this state, which is progressively attenuated, generally lasts 5 to 10 times as long as the absolute refractory period (and action potential). It is sometimes followed, due to 'overswing' of the restorative mechanism, by a short period of hyperexcitability.

The action potential, as opposed to the post-synaptic or end-plate potential, is said to be an **all-or-nothing** phenomenon. That is to say, either the membrane is sufficiently depolarized to initiate a propagated action potential, or it isn't. But this does not mean that in any given axon, that the size (i.e. voltage) or rate of propagation of the action potential* is always constant. It will be so for constant conditions of the membrane; but when the membrane is altered, as in the relative refractory period, both the amplitude and conduction velocity of the spike are reduced. Because of this, an axon which can conduct a single action potential with a duration (and absolute refractory period) of o·5 ms, is not able in fact to conduct impulses at the rate of 2000/sec, but has an upper limit of about 1000/sec.

* The action potential in a single nerve fibre is usually recorded on a short time basis, so that it looks like, and is called, **a spike** (Fig. 13).

At (striated) neuromuscular junctions in mammals, the transmitter substance is always excitatory. But at neuroneuronal contacts in the central nervous system, not only do E-substances occur, but in some cases an inhibitory transmitter, or I-substance, is found. Here as for E-substances, several chemical substances are known to be involved. Whatever their chemical nature, I-substances, when released from appropriate axon terminals on to a post-synaptic membrane, have a hyperpolarizing effect on the latter, which increases its impermeability. Consider, for example, a neurone in which the resting membrane potential is 70 mV and in which an action potential is generated when the membrane potential falls to 60 mV; in such a neurone the effect of I-substance might be to increase the membrane potential to 90 mV. It would then be necessary to depolarize (excite) by 30 mV, instead of 10 mV, to the critical firing point of 60 mV.

Like E-substance, I-substance is destroyed by an enzyme, so that the hyperpolarization which it causes is of short duration. For inhibition to occur under physiological conditions, it is evident that the hyperpolarizing effect must take place, and be present, *before* the arrival of the depolarizing impulse which would normally excite the membrane. This type of inhibition is called **post-synaptic**, because the effect is on a post-synaptic membrane. It could obviously be overcome if the excitatory (depolarizing) effect were great enough.

By current theories, the neurone doctrine makes it inconceivable that some terminals of a given axon could liberate E-substance and others I-substance; there must be separate excitatory and inhibitory neurones, all of whose terminals liberate E- and I-substance respectively. It is generally accepted that an inhibitory pathway, upon being sufficiently excited by E-substance, generates an action potential which is conducted along its axon and causes the liberation of I-substances at its terminals. A good example of this is the self-inhibition of motoneurone activity by the Renshaw mechanism (Fig. 19, Chapter 6).

Another type of inhibition has been demonstrated, which was thought to be due to axo-axonal (termino-terminal) synaptic contacts, and so is called **pre-synaptic inhibition**. It now seems likely that the morphological basis of this type of inhibition is the vesicle-containing process of an inhibitory interneurone (Chapter 2) taking part in a synaptic glomerulus; an excitatory afferent activates the interneuronal process, which in its turn inhibits a relay neurone (Fig. 4). It should be noted that some excitatory terminals synapse directly with the relay neurone, producing normal excitation; it is only when an interneuronal process is interposed between the two that 'presynaptic' inhibition occurs. The mechanism of presynaptic inhibition consists of the reduction of the quantity of excitatory transmitter substance released from the inhibited axon terminal.

It may be useful to tabulate some of the contrasting characteristics of pre- and post-synaptic inhibition:

	Pre-synaptic inhibition	*Post-synaptic inhibition*
Average latency	long	short
Average duration	long	short
Effect of strychnine	None	Abolishes or greatly depresses

Classification of Neurones

The essential part of a neurone consists of a cable-like structure (the axon) along which a self-propagating action potential can pass. At one end of this axon are receptive filaments, the dendrites, while at the other end are transmitting filaments, the axon terminals. The nerve cell body (responsible for the metabolism of the neurone) may be intercalated at any point in this longitudinal structure, or on a side-branch from it (Fig. 2).

Morphological classification can be made on the basis of the axon, in two ways which are of physiological significance:

1. Whether the axon has a large or small number of collateral branches. In general, primitive (phylogenetically ancient) iso-dendritic neurone systems tend to be made up of neurones whose

axons have many collateral branches, while phylogenetically recent tufted neurone systems have axons with few collaterals. This classification is of importance in the consideration of system physiology within the central nervous system (Chapter 2).

2. Axon diameter, and whether or not the axis cylinder is enclosed in a noded myelin sheath. These factors affect conduction velocity; and, happily for the student, myelinated neurones with particular diameters and conduction velocities seem to be associated with particular functions in the peripheral nervous system. However, note must be taken straightaway that a considerable degree of overlap exists (vide infra).

Peripheral fibres were first classified, according to their properties and location, into groups A, B, and C; these will be considered in reverse order.

C fibres consist of all 'unmyelinated' axons. They have diameters from considerably less than 1μm up to 2μm, and conduction velocities from 0·7–2 metres/sec. They are also known as Group IV fibres.

B fibres are myelinated, but are peculiar to the preganglionic neurones of the autonomic nervous system of mammals. They have a diameter of about 3μm, with conduction velocities varying from 3–5 metres/sec. They are said to differ from other myelinated axons in having an action potential of rather longer duration (1·2 ms, as against 0·5 ms).

All other myelinated axons with nodes of Ranvier fall into the A group. In descending order of conduction velocity, A fibres have been further divided into subgroups α, β, γ and δ.

Workers researching on peripheral muscular **afferent** fibres have evolved a different classification, in which the Roman numerals I to IV are used, again in descending order of conduction velocity. As has been noted above, Group IV corresponds to C fibres. Unfortunately Groups I to III have no exact correspondence with the subgroups α, β, γ and δ of the A group. Confusion is therefore best avoided if the alphabetical grouping is restricted to efferent and cutaneous fibres, and the numerical one to muscular afferent fibres, as in the Table below.

Classification of Myelinated Peripheral Axons

Class		Destination or origin	Diameter μm	Velocity m/sec
Motor	α	Extrafusal muscle fibres	12–18	60–100
fibres	γ	Intrafusal muscle fibres	2–8	10–30
Deep afferents	I	Primary muscle and tendon receptors	12–22	70–120
	II	Secondary muscle receptors	6–12	30–70
	III	Aponeuroses, joints, 'deep' pain receptors	2–6	12–30
Cutaneous	α, β	Tactile receptors	6–12	30–70
afferents	γ, δ	Head, cold 'fast' pain	2–6	12–30

CHAPTER FIVE

Receptors and Effectors

Receptors are essentially **transducers**; that is to say, they turn forms of energy into nerve impulses (i.e. nervous energy). Most receptors are specific, in that they typically transmute one particular form of energy, although they may also respond to other forms of energy at high intensity and their activity sometimes varies with body temperature.

Receptors may be classified in several ways:

1. By site of receptors. **Exteroceptors** react to forms of energy external to the body (light energy → vision; sound energy → audition; chemical energy → smell and taste; mechanical energy → touch, pressure, etc; thermal energy → heat and cold). **Proprioceptors** respond to variations of mechanical energy within muscles, tendons, and joints and **enteroceptors** to forms of energy acting on the viscera.

2. By site of action of the physical energy concerned. Thus the **special senses** are concerned with events transmitted to various cranial nerves by the appropriate special sense organs; the **superficial senses** are concerned with events occurring in the skin and subjacent tissues; the **deep senses** with those taking place in the deep tissues.

3. By fibre diameter.

These classifications are however either partly physical (depending on the form of physical energy concerned) or anatomical (depending on the location of the receptors). A slightly more physiological classification is given in the Table, Chapter 4, where modality specificity is related (within the myelinated or A group of fibres) to the diameter of the fibre and hence to conduction velocity. However, account must be taken of the fact that all forms of energy acting on the surface of the body (thermal, chemical and mechanical) are also able to evoke activity in primary afferent fibres of the C (Group IV) or unmyelinated group at high intensities. Such fibres, distributed in deep tissues as well as in the tegument, signal tissue damage (pain), and are known as **polymodal nociceptors.**

Primary afferent neurones may be regarded as having the nerve cell body displaced centripetally along the axon, so that the (often myelinated) fibres conducting towards the cell body is a part of the axon, as well as the portion leading from the cell body into the central nervous system (Fig. 2). Thus the peripheral unmyelinated terminal filaments (or filament) function in the same way as the dendrites of a neurone within the central nervous system. Only the central terminals are true telodendria, and bear synaptic knobs. The peripheral terminals of primary afferent nerve fibres may end in one of two ways. They may be in contact with a specific receptor cell (e.g. the photoreceptors of the retina) or organule (e.g. Pacini corpuscles), or they may ramify apparently freely in the skin. Between these two extremes lie those cutaneous nerve fibres whose terminals end in association with ill-defined epidermal structures. Some of these have been named and de-scribed, but it is recognized that many intermediate forms exist. In view of this confusion, it has even been doubted whether any truly 'free' nerve terminals exist. The complex consisting of the receptor cells, if non-neural, and associated primary afferent neurone is known as a **sensory unit** (cf. **motor unit,** p. 41). Whatever the structures involved, there is no doubt as to the punctate nature of cutaneous sensibility in man; spots can be found sensitive only to touch, pressure, heat, cold, or pain.* Thus while primary afferent fibres fired by all modalities of sensation have been studied, it has only been possible so far to investigate those receptors whose structure and physical sensitivity are clearly defined.

---

* At least some sorts of pain are produced by tissue damage. In such a case the receptors are probably activated by chemical substances liberated by tissue breakdown, however this is initially produced.

At physiological intensities of stimulation, receptors (and this includes 'free' nerve terminals, if they exist) transduce only one form of physical energy and thus are **modality specific**. This transduction is effected in one of two ways. The application of the appropriate form of physical energy to the receptor causes it either to secrete a chemical transmitter substance onto its associated nerve terminal, or to build up a potential difference within itself. In the latter case, this is known as the **receptor potential**. The effect of either the chemical transmitter or the receptor potential is to induce a potential change in the peripheral terminal filaments of the primary afferent nerve. This nerve potential is in every way similar to the post-synaptic potential discussed in the preceding chapter: it is called the **generator potential**. If the generator potential is sufficiently large, it will fire off an all-or-none action potential in the nerve fibre. Note that in the case where the nerve terminal is itself the receptor, the receptor and generator potentials are one and the same thing.

The Pacini corpuscle has been carefully studied, and it is known that the action potential arises at the first node of Ranvier (which is outside the actual corpuscle). It is also known that each Pacini corpuscle is innervated by a separate axon, so that in this case there is a one-to-one relationship between receptor and nerve fibre, and a single receptor is capable of producing a sufficiently large receptor potential to generate a sufficiently large generator potential to fire the axon. However, the vast majority of receptors show the important phenomenon of **convergence**. Thus, for example, while there are over 100 million photoreceptors (rods and cones) in the human retina, there are only 1 million optic nerve fibres. The number of intercalated bipolar cells is somewhere in between these two figures, but it is evident that a large number of receptor units converge on each bipolar cell; and many bipolar cells converge on each ganglion cell (outside the macula). Similarly, in the case of many primary afferent nerve fibres, spatial summation from a number of receptor units is probably necessary to produce sufficient depolarization to fire off an action potential.

Three important general properties of sensory units (consisting of receptors and their associated nerve fibres) should now be considered. These are:

1. **Threshold**, which may be defined as the minimum quantity of appropriate physical energy required to set up a propagated action potential in a primary afferent nerve. Many receptors are exquisitely sensitive; for example a Pacini corpuscle fires its axon in response to a deformation of 0·5 μm maintained for 0·1 sec. In the case of convergence of receptors on single axons, some idea of threshold may be gained by measuring the minimal quantities of energy required to provoke conscious sensation in human subjects. Thus the human eye (under optimal atmospheric conditions) is said to be able to perceive the light from a single candle 28 miles away; a sensation of cold is felt if the skin temperature be lowered 1·0°C for 3 sec, or of warmth if the skin temperature is raised 0·03°C for 3 sec. On the other hand, some receptors have a relatively high threshold, such as pricking receptors, or even polymodal nociceptors (page 37) at the highest end. When considering the latter, **sensory threshold** for pain, which varies very little from one individual to another, should not be confused with the **tolerance level** for pain, which varies enormously between cultures, between individuals, and even within the same individual at different times.

2. **Frequency Coding.** Within the working range of physiological usefulness of any given receptor and its associated nerve fibre, there is a direct relationship between the intensity of the applied stimulus and the frequency of the impulses passing up the nerve. Thus at low (but supraliminal) intensities of stimulation, only one or a few impulses will be transmitted along the nerve in unit time, whereas at successively high intensities a progressively larger number of nervous impulses will be initiated in the same unit time.

3. **Adaptation.** Some receptors (called slowly adapting or tonic) may continue to generate nervous impulses for as long as they are subjected to the appropriate physical force, i.e. so long as the adequate stimulus is maintained. The supreme example of this type of receptor is the flower-spray (secondary) receptor of the intrafusal muscle spindle. Other receptors (called rapidly adapting or phasic), on the other hand, generate nervous impulses

when a stimulus is applied, but cease to do so if the stimulus is maintained; it should be noted, however, that some such receptors may generate another burst of impulses when the stimulus is removed, i.e. in this case they transduce an 'off' as well as an 'on' effect. The Pacini corpuscle is an example of a rapidly adapting receptor. In physical terms, slowly adapting receptors may be said to signal steady state, while rapidly adapting ones signal change of state.

Receptors adapt with varying rapidity, so that there is a whole range of adaptability as a function of time with regard to different receptors. Interesting intermediate forms occur, such as many receptors in and around joint capsules. Their axons may show a steady 'background' discharge when the joint is at rest, while movement evokes acceleration or deceleration of the resting discharge rate. If the changed rate of discharge is maintained after the movement has ceased and the joint is in a new position, it is slowly adapting, and obviously the rate of discharge from such a receptor signals the position of the joint; if on the other hand the rate of discharge returns to its former level after the movement is over, the receptor is rapidly adapting and evidently signals rate of movement.

Some receptors can be 'set' by the central nervous system. The classical example of this is the muscle spindle organ. The tension of the intrafusal muscle fibre containing the spindle organ is controlled by γ efferent motor fibres, whose cells of origin lie in the ventral horn of the spinal cord. By causing the intrafusal muscle fibre to contract, the centrally-operated γ motor neurone can increase the discharge rate in the afferent axon coming from the spindle receptor in the same muscle fibre. The Group I afferent, the γ efferent, and the intrafusal muscle fibre are often referred to as the γ-loop. More recently some efferent controls on other receptors have been described; for example it has been shown that neurones in the superior olivary nucleus of the cat send axons to the acoustic hair cells of the cochlea (olivo-cochlear bundle) which modify the discharge rate of fibres coming from the cochlear receptors. Efferents to the retina have been demonstrated in birds, and may have a similar function.

It should be noted that, in vertebrates, peripheral 'synapses', consisting of junctions between receptors and primary afferent fibres, and junctions between efferent axons and striated muscles, are purely excitatory. However, some junctions between peripheral autonomic fibres and the muscles they innervate may be inhibitory, although most are excitatory. Some inhibitory effects can also be obtained by peripheral receptor stimulation, but these are due to synaptic arrangements at the first relay in the central nervous system, as will be explained in later chapters.

Lastly, it is important to distinguish between **afferent** and **sensory**. Conscious sensation is a property of the central nervous system, and is in no way dependent on receptors as such, but only on their connections within the central nervous system.

Effectors are muscles and glands. As explained in Chapter 4, striated muscle fibres are universally excited by the arrival of nervous impulses. Smooth and cardiac muscles and glands are controlled by the autonomic nervous system, and their neuro-muscular or neuroglandular 'synapses' appear to be of a very simple type. It should be noted, however, that heart muscle and the smooth muscle of the gastro-intestinal tract are not paralysed by denervation, as is striated muscle; they exhibit intrinsic activity, which is modified rather than initiated by nervous control.

Glands also may respond, under physiological conditions, to direct stimulation, without the intervention of nervous control, as occurs in the intestine. When glandular secretion is brought about by nervous stimulation, it may vary in chemical composition according to whether the nervous impulses originate in the sympathetic or parasympathetic divisions of the autonomic nervous system.

The neuromuscular synapses (motor end plates) between somatic motor nerve fibres and striated muscle fibres have already been described. We must now introduce the important concept of the **motor unit**. This is defined as the number of muscle fibres innervated, and therefore controlled, by a single nerve fibre. Such a unit acts as an entity—either all of its fibres contract maximally, or none of them contract. Any given muscle is made up of a number of motor units, and the strength of contraction of the muscle as a whole depends upon how many of its motor units are activated. The duration of the action potential (and hence of the absolute and relative refractory periods) of striated muscle fibres is longer than that of the myelinated nerve fibres which supply them; thus repetitive impulses can be discharged along the nerve faster than the muscle fibres can cope with them, so ensuring that the muscle fibres can be kept in a state of constant and smooth contraction. However, such tetanic contraction of a single motor unit rapidly brings about fatigue of the muscle fibres. Under normal circumstances, smooth contraction of a muscle as a whole is brought about by less rapid (subtetanic) but asynchronous activity of all its motor units. This means that while individual units are alternately contracting and relaxing, the fact that they are out of phase with one another ensures that the contraction of the whole muscle will be smoothly maintained.

The size of motor units is of the greatest importance. The numbers of muscle fibres innervated by a single motor axon varies from about 5 (in the external ocular muscles) to about 1500 (in the proximal limb muscles). In the ultimate analysis, muscular 'skill' depends on the smallness of motor units, and this in turn will depend on the number of motoneurones available to supply a given bulk of muscle. Thus, for example, human superiority in manual dexterity over other primates may be due to smaller motor units in the muscles acting on the human hand.

The Spinal Cord

The spinal cord shows a simpler arrangement than the brain, but if the basic pattern of its morphology be properly understood, the higher centres of the CNS can be seen as more complicated variations on the same theme.

The spinal cord extends from the foramen magnum to the second lumbar vertebra, and its lower end is tethered to the back of the coccyx by the filum terminale. Some thirty-two pairs of spinal nerves emerge from the cord and pass downwards to make their exit from the intervertebral foramina. Due to the relative shortness of the cord compared with the vertebral column the downward direction of the nerves is very marked in the lower part of the vertebral canal, and the leash of nerves below the lower part of the cord is known as the **cauda equina**. Those parts of the cord from which the large nerves of the brachial and lumbo-sacral plexuses arise can be seen on gross inspection to be swollen relative to the parts immediately above and below; these are called the **cervical** and **lumbar enlargements**.

A transverse section of the spinal cord reveals the central grey core to be arranged in a butterfly shape. The wings are referred to as **posterior** or **dorsal** and **anterior** or **ventral** horns (Fig. 16). There is an (anterior median) sulcus in the white matter, which does not reach so far centrally as the grey matter, so that nerve fibres can cross ventral to it from one side of the cord to the other, in the **anterior white commissure**. While there is no sulcus in the posterior or dorsal aspect of the cord, there is a (posterior median) septum which reaches as far centrally as the grey matter, so that there is no posterior white commissure.

The shape of the grey core naturally divides the white matter into columns or funiculi. The posterior horns reach the surface

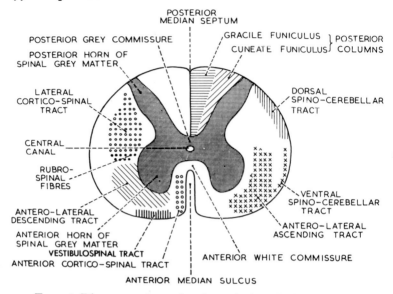

POSTERIOR
MEDIAN SEPTUM

POSTERIOR GREY COMMISSURE

GRACILE FUNICULUS ⎱ POSTERIOR
CUNEATE FUNICULUS ⎰ COLUMNS

POSTERIOR HORN OF
SPINAL GREY MATTER

LATERAL
CORTICO-SPINAL
TRACT

DORSAL
SPINO-CEREBELLAR
TRACT

CENTRAL
CANAL

RUBRO-
SPINAL
FIBRES

VENTRAL
SPINO-CEREBELLAR
TRACT

ANTERO-LATERAL
DESCENDING TRACT

ANTERO-LATERAL
ASCENDING TRACT

ANTERIOR HORN OF
SPINAL GREY MATTER

VESTIBULOSPINAL TRACT

ANTERIOR CORTICO-SPINAL TRACT

ANTERIOR WHITE COMMISSURE

ANTERIOR MEDIAN SULCUS

FIG. 16. Diagrammatic section through the spinal cord. Long
ascending fibres are shown on the right, descending on the
left.

of the cord, and the white matter between the posterior horns of
the two sides form the **posterior** or **dorsal columns**. The
anterior horns do not reach the surface, but the **anterior funiculi**
lie between them, imperfectly divided off from the **lateral
columns** which lie between the anterior and posterior horns. It is
usual to divide the lateral columns into anterolateral and postero-
lateral parts.

A large number of the white fibres in the cord are either
descending from the brain to lower centres in the cord, or ascending from the cord to higher centres in the brain. It is therefore
obvious that the amount of white matter in the cord is greatest at
high cervical levels and least at sacral. The grey matter on the
other hand is a continuous core of cells which varies in amount
at different levels. It is greatest in amount at the levels where the
largest nerve roots leave or join the cord, i.e. at the cervical and
lumbar enlargements.

The dorsal columns (gracile and cuneate funiculi) contain long
collaterals of $A\beta$ primary afferent fibres coming from cutaneous

mechanoreceptors and Aβ stem fibres coming from articular mechanoreceptors. Ascending on the periphery of the lateral white column are, dorsally, the **dorsal spinocerebellar tract** and ventrally the **ventral spinocerebellar tract.** Deeper in the anterolateral white matter are found ascending **spinoreticular** and **spinothalamic** fibres. Note that the dorsal columns and dorsal spinocerebellar tract are ipsilateral with respect to the side from which their peripheral input is derived, while the ventral spinocerebellar and spinothalamic pathways are crossed; spinoreticular fibres are both crossed and uncrossed.

Long descending fibres are found only in the lateral and anterior funiculi. From dorsal to ventral (Fig. 16) they are: (a) the (crossed) **corticospinal (pyramidal) tract,** coming from the sensorimotor cortex; (b) the (crossed) **rubrospinal tract** from the red nucleus in the midbrain; (c) (crossed and uncrossed) **reticulospinal fibres** from the pontine and medullary reticular formation; (d) (uncrossed) **vestibulospinal fibres** from the lateral vestibular nucleus of the medulla oblongata. It may be observed

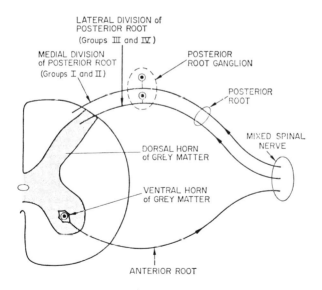

FIG. 17. The anterior (ventral) and posterior (dorsal) roots of a mixed spinal nerve.

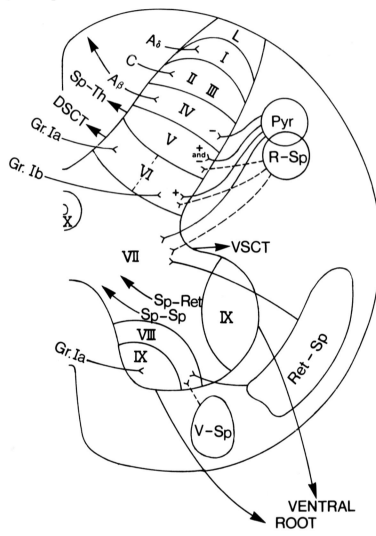

FIG. 18. Schematic diagram of the spinal cord laminae. The peripheral afferent input (Group I and Aβ, Aδ and C fibres) from the dorsal roots is shown on the left; note that collaterals from Aβ primary afferents pass directly into the dorsal columns. L = Tract of Lissauer; Pyr = Pyramidal Tract; R-Sp. = Rubrospinal fibres; Ret-Sp. = Reticulospinal fibres; V-Sp. = Vestibulospinal fibres. + and/or − indicate excitatory or inhibitory effects of pyramidal neurones. (Some

from Fig. 18 that descending fibres terminate in those grey laminae to which they are most closely placed.

It should be noted that, apart from the dorsal columns, none of the 'tracts' in the spinal white matter are pure; they are all mixed with other ascending and descending fibres.

With this basic information the fundamental arrangement of the spinal cord and its nerves can be studied. Every spinal nerve has a **dorsal** (sensory) and **ventral** (motor) **root** (Fig. 17). The ventral roots consist of axons given off by anterior horn cells; these emerge as discrete clumps of fibres which are gathered together as the root. At its exit from the dura, the fibres of the ventral root join those of the dorsal root to form a mixed (motor and sensory) nerve. The anterior horn cells of the cord are represented in the brain stem by the nuclei of the somatic efferent columns (cranial nerves, III, IV, VI, XII). Between the first thoracic and second lumbar segments of the cord, and again in the second, third and fourth sacral segments, some motor cells, smaller than those in the anterior horn, are found in the lateral part of the spinal grey (intermediolateral cell column). These give rise to axons which emerge with the ventral root and are distributed (T1–L2) as **white rami communicantes** to the ganglia of the sympathetic chain, or to the pelvic autonomic (parasympathetic) ganglia (S2, 3, 4). The intermediolateral grey column is represented in the brain stem by the dorsal motor nucleus of the vagus, the salivatory nuclei, and the Edinger–Westphal nucleus of the oculomotor nerve.

The fibres of the dorsal root conduct impulses from the periphery **towards** the cell body. The primary afferent nerve cell bodies are to be found in the dorsal root ganglia, which are encapsulated collections of nerve cells lying in a pocket of dura just central to the point at which the ventral and dorsal roots join. Their axons enter the tip of the posterior horn as a large-fibred

---

lines are interrupted purely to avoid confusion with nearby solid lines.) DSCT, VSCT = Dorsal and ventral spino-cerebellar tracts; Sp-Th. = Spinothalamic fibres; Sp-Ret. = Spinoreticular fibres; Sp-Sp. = Spinospinal fibres.

medial division containing fibres of groups I and II (Aβ) (from various mechanoreceptors only), which actually enters medial to the grey matter, and a small fibred **lateral division** containing fibres from groups Aδ and C (which also include some mechanoreceptor afferents as well as those from receptors of other modalities) which penetrates the grey matter (Fig. 17). Examination of the spinal cord will reveal the posterior root fibres to enter the cord in a continuous row rather than in clumps, as do the anterior roots.

The grey matter of the spinal cord is divided into a number of functionally and morphologically distinct laminae, represented by Roman numerals beginning at the extremity of the posterior horn (Fig. 18). These laminae contain the cell bodies of functionally discrete neurones, but it is important to note that in some instances, dendrites spread into other laminae.

Lamina I constitutes the marginal zone and receives small myelinated (Aδ, Group III) primary afferents, while layers II (and III, according to some authorities), at the top of the dorsal horn, make up the **substantia gelatinosa**. It is made up of small cells whose axons run up or down a few segments of the cord, as the **tract of Lissauer,** to synapse with other regions of the substantia gelatinosa and of inhibitory Golgi type II interneurones. Axon collaterals within the substantia gelatinosa engage dendrites of cells from the underlying lamina IV, which spread out into lamina III. Unmyelinated primary afferents (Group C or IV) in dorsal roots terminate in synaptic contact with gelatinosal cells. They carry impulses from high-threshold mechanoreceptors and other sensory modalities represented in the unmyelinated fibre spectrum.

Lamina IV consists of neurones which receive primary afferents of Aβ fibres coming from cutaneous mechanoreceptors; collaterals of these incoming fibres join with primary afferents from joints to pass up the dorsal columns as the gracile and cuneate funiculi. In addition to excitation by cutaneous Aβ primary afferents, the activity of lamina IV cells is modulated by gelatinosal cells receiving unmyelinated primary afferents. The descending fibres of the corticospinal tract exert an inhibitory influence on the cells of lamina IV. The cells of lamina V receive a convergent input from lamina IV, and their axons, in their turn, converge on neurones in lamina VI; long collaterals of lamina V axons together with some efferents from lamina I form (neo)**spinothalamic fibres** which pass upwards in the anterolateral columns of the opposite side of the spinal cord; they cross obliquely and take some five or six segments to reach the anterolateral quadrant of the opposite side of the cord. Descending corticospinal fibres have both excitatory and inhibitory effects on lamina V, and rubrospinal fibres also exert an influence here.

Lamina VI, at the base of the dorsal horn, is divided into medial and lateral parts. The large Group Ia primary afferents from muscle spindles synapse with the cells of the medial part of lamina VI, known as the **Column of Clarke** between the second lumbar and mid-cervical segments, where its cells are particularly large, while a primary afferent collateral goes on to innervate directly the α motoneurones of lamina IX. Efferent fibres from medial lamina VI form the dorsal spinocerebellar tract, which passes up the periphery of the dorsal part of the ipsilateral lateral white column. The neurones of the lateral part of lamina VI, in addition to receiving a convergent input from lamina V, receive the peripheral afferent Ib fibres coming from Golgi tendon organs, and send its efferents across the spinal cord to ascend on the periphery of the ventral part of the contralateral white column as the ventral spinocerebellar tract. Cells of lamina VI also project to deeper laminae of the spinal grey matter, perhaps including the moto-neurone lamina IX. Long descending fibres ending in lamina VI include the rubrospinal tract and the corticospinal tract (which has an excitatory effect on this lamina).

Laminae VII and VIII abut directly on the motoneurone lamina IX, as well as upon the central lamina X surrounding the central canal. In addition to the cell bodies of those neurones proper to the laminae themselves, they also contain motoneurone dendrites from lamina IX. Laminae VII and VIII receive no direct peripheral input, but there is a powerful convergent input from some of the more dorsally-placed laminae which do receive peripheral afferents. These neurones are also influenced from the other side of the spinal cord, probably through lamina X. Descending reticulospinal fibres end in laminae VII and VIII, and vestibulospinal fibres in lamina VIII. At least some of these fibres must end in contact with motoneurone dendrites, for monosynaptic effects of these pathways have been demonstrated on motoneurones. Efferents from lamina VII certainly travel for varying distances up and down the spinal cord to synapse with lamina VII cells at other levels, for intersegmental effects can be recorded in lamina VII; longer axons reach the brainstem as spinoreticular fibres, and certainly lamina VII, and perhaps also lamina VIII, should be regarded as the spinal component of the reticular formation (q.v.).

The motoneurones whose axons pass out of the spinal cord as ventral roots constitute lamina IX. Motoneurones are grouped according to whether they supply axial or limb musculature, flexors or extensors. They are of two kinds, large α motoneurones which supply extrafusal muscle fibres and smaller γ motoneurones which supply intrafusal muscle fibres, which contain the spindle apparatus. It has already been mentioned that motoneurone dendrites spread into adjacent laminae where they come into synaptic contact with vestibulospinal and reticulospinal fibres. In lamina IX itself, α motoneurones receive a direct primary afferent supply from collaterals of Ia fibres coming from muscle spindles. These form the basis of the **monosynaptic segmental reflex arc**, which is responsible for the various 'jerk' reflexes—elbow, wrist, knee, ankle, etc. In the cervical, and perhaps the lumbar, enlargements, motoneurones concerned with movements of the digits are directly contacted by corticospinal fibres. However, it should be noted that for the most part, corticospinal influence on motoneurones is indirect, occurring through interneurones in laminae IV, V and VI.

Information about the spinal grey matter and its connections are summarized in the table on p. 52.

The anterior horn cell and its axon, which emerges as the ventral root of the mixed spinal nerve, are known clinically as the **lower motor neurone**. It is the final common pathway whereby motor impulses are transmitted to effector organs (usually muscles). Thus a lesion of the lower motor neurone leads to a complete paralysis of the structure innervated. A muscle deprived of its lower motor neurone innervation becomes completely **flaccid**, and wastes away. The long descending fibres whose impulses influence the activity of anterior horn cells, are collectively known as the **upper motor neurone**. If these are damaged, the lower motor neurone is unable to receive and transmit certain impulses, particularly those subserving voluntary (willed) movement; this condition is known as **paresis**. On the other hand, descending inhibitory influences are also removed so that the anterior horn cells discharge more than usually into the muscles; so instead of flaccidity, there is a condition of increased tone known as **spasticity**. The segmental monosynaptic arcs are of course unaffected in an upper motor neurone lesion, so the reflexes are intact (they are often increased, because of the removal of descending inhibitory influences).

It will be seen that although a number of long ascending and descending 'tracts' in the spinal cord are named, none of them (except possibly the posterior columns) occupy a discrete area of the white matter. The fibres of all of them are to a certain extent mixed with those of other ascending and descending systems, and probably to a much larger extent with ascending and descending spino-spinal axons.

The spinal cord represents the lowest, that is to say the most primitive, level of the central nervous system. Even so, it presents a high degree of organization, and its physiological characteristics are very far from being wholly elucidated. When the spinal cord is separated from the higher parts of the central nervous system, it is at first almost entirely inert—a condition known as **spinal shock**. In general, the duration of spinal shock is dependent on the degree of supraspinal (cerebral) control. Thus it is shortest in the lower vertebrates and longest in the highest primates. When the phase of spinal shock is over, the cord shows a certain degree of independent function. Comparison of results from experiments conducted on intact and spinal animals make it possible to separate the **intrinsic activity** of the spinal cord, and its modification by supraspinal (descending) control. Some of the intrinsic properties of the spinal cord will be described here, and

Receptor	Primary afferent fibres	Descending afferent fibres	Lamina	Extrasegmental efferent fibres	Intra-segmental projections
High-threshold mechanoreceptors and thermoreceptors	Aδ (Group III)		I (Marginal zone)	Spinothalamic (to thalamus)	Deeper Laminae
Polymodal nociceptors	Unmyelinated (Group IV or C)		II, (III) (Substantia gelatinosa cells and lamina IV dendrites)	Tract of Lissauer (to other regions of substantia gelatinosa)	Lamina IV dendrites
Cutaneous mechanoreceptors Aβ	(Group II)	Corticospinal (−)	IV	Spinothalamic (to Thalamus)	Lamina V
		Corticospinal (+ and −) Rubrospinal	V		Laminae IV and VII
Muscle spindles	Group Ia	Corticospinal (+) and Rubrospinal	VI (medial)	Dorsal spinocerebellar tract (to Cerebellum)	
Golgi tendon organs	Group Ib		VI (lateral)	Ventral spinocerebellar tract (to Cerebellum)	Lamina IX
		Corticospinal Rubrospinal Reticulospinal (+ and −) Vestibulospinal (+)	VII and VIII cells and lamina IX dendrites	Spinospinal and spinoreticular (to other regions of lamina VII, brainstem reticular formation)	Laminae VII and IX
Muscle spindles	Group Ia (collaterals to α motoneurones only)	Corticospinal to segments controlling movement of digits	IX (α and γ motoneurones)	Ventral roots (to effectors)	

subsequently their modification by control from higher centres in later chapters.

The intrinsic mechanisms, classically described as spinal, are in fact segmental. They can occur at any level of the neuraxis which has a (primary afferent) inflow from the periphery and a (primary efferent) outflow to effector organs; they are therefore found not only in the spinal cord, but also in those parts of the brain stem which contain cranial nerve nuclei.

Intrinsic Spinal Mechanisms

THE MONOSYNAPTIC (STRETCH OR MYOTACTIC) REFLEX

Although this is the simplest reflex mechanism, it is probably fairly sophisticated from an evolutionary point of view, as large fibres with restricted terminations represent a recent development.

Basically (Fig. 19) the reflex depends upon the fact that Group Ia primary afferent fibres coming from spindle organs in intrafusal muscle fibres send an axon branch to the α-motoneurones which innervate the extrafusal fibres of the same muscle. Thus, when the muscle fibres are suddenly elongated (stretched), as by a tap with a patellar hammer on a tendon, the spindle organs discharge into the afferent fibres, which fire the α-motoneurones. This causes the extrafusal muscle fibres to contract, thus restoring the muscle to its original length.

It must not be imagined that the stretch reflex is evoked only when a muscle is artificially lengthened by an examiner. In fact it comes into play whenever there is a change in the length of a muscle. Moreover, it is only in its simplest form that the reflex is monosynaptic. Because of the profusion of axon collaterals and terminals, alternative pathways involving more than one synapse are available. Nor indeed is the reflex, in the intact living animal, necessarily limited to one segment of the neuraxis, for two reasons: (i) The terminal branches of a single peripheral afferent fibre may be distributed over several segments, and (ii) the change in length of one neuromuscular unit will bring about changes in other units within the same muscle, and even in other muscles alto-gether, so that a sort of chain reaction may occur involving whole groups of muscles with their afferent and efferent neurones.

Even in its simplest form, the stretch reflex illustrates an important principle of central nervous activity as a whole. This is the principle of **homeostasis**, whereby the central nervous system acts as a homeostat to restore the status quo of the organism.

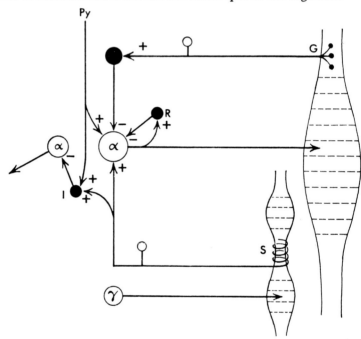

FIG. 19. α motoneurones innervate striated muscle, while an axon collateral excites a Renshaw cell (R), which recurrently inhibits the motoneurone. The α cells may be excited by fibres of the pyramidal tract (Py), and by primary afferents coming from spindles (S) in intrafusal muscle fibres supplied by γ motoneurones, but both of these sources may also excite an inhibitory interneurone (I) which inhibits the α moto-neurones supplying antagonistic muscles. Primary afferents coming from Golgi tendon organs (G) also excite an inhibitory interneurone which inhibits the α motoneurone supplying the muscle which acts through the tendon.

Because muscle stretch receptors are slowly adapting, they would, in the absence of other mechanisms, continue to fire the α-motoneurones for as long as the length of the muscle is changing; and this might cause the motoneurones greatly to overcompensate. This is to some extent prevented by the following inhibitory mechanisms:

RECURRENT INHIBITION (FIG. 19)

In this mechanism, an intraspinal axon collateral of the moto-neurone fires an interneurone. This interneurone, known as a Renshaw cell, sends its short axon back to the motoneurone. The Renshaw cell is an inhibitory neurone, so that, when excited, its axon terminals hyperpolarize the membrane of the motoneurone, thus inhibiting its activity—or, to be exact, raising its threshold of excitability. Recurrent inhibition of motoneurones does not only occur during the course of the stretch reflex, but obviously comes into play whatever the means by which the α-motoneurones are excited.

DISYNAPTIC INHIBITION (FIG. 19)

Group Ib afferents coming from Golgi tendon organs establish synaptic contact with an inhibitory interneurone in the spinal grey matter, whose axon impinges on the α-motoneurone supply-ing extrafusal muscle fibres acting on the same tendon.

RECIPROCAL INHIBITION (FIG. 19)

This represents a further modification of the stretch reflex, still occurring at the level of a single spinal cord segment. In this case, we are dealing with the connections of a second collateral branch of the primary afferent fibre coming from the stretch receptor. This second collateral excites an inhibitory interneurone, which hyperpolarizes motoneurones supplying muscles antagonistic to that which is contracting as a result of the stretch reflex.

Again, it must not be imagined that the inhibitory interneurone concerned in reciprocal inhibition is fired only by Group 1 primary afferents; indeed it is only recently that this has been demonstrated. The principle of reciprocal inhibition was described by Sherrington in connection with impulses descending from higher levels; thus excitation (contraction) of a muscle brought about by stimulation of the corticospinal tract is accompanied by inhibition of its antagonists, and there is no reason to believe that the same inhibitory interneurone should not be involved.

POSITIVE SUPPORTING REACTIONS

Light pressure on the sole (pad) of the foot or slight stretching of the interosseous muscles, activating low threshold (Aβ) cutaneous and muscle receptors respectively, cause reflex contraction of all the extensor muscles of the limb, such that it tends to maintain contact with the stimulating surface.* This reflex is intersegmental rather than segmental; for the afferent impulses are coming only from those dorsal roots supplying the extremity of the limb, while the efferent outflow to extensor muscles also comes from ventral horn cells in segments rostral to that stimulated.

The positive supporting reactions illustrate that there is a built-in, genetic, difference between the connections (and therefore the reactions) of flexor and extensor motoneurones. It is of course the limb and neck extensor muscles which are in play during the maintenance of normal posture. By the same token, reflex activity in response to the low threshold stimuli differs according to whether the stimulus is applied to parts of the body which are or are not normally weight-bearing. Under suitable experimental conditions, a spinal animal placed on its side on a horizontal surface will struggle to adopt the normal standing position. This comes about by the interaction of a whole series of positive (and perhaps converse negative) supporting reactions.

* The **plantar reflex,** so important in clinical neurology, belongs to the general category of positive supporting reactions, but differs in being under supraspinal (pyramidal) control.

THE WITHDRAWAL REFLEX

In contrast to the supporting reaction described above, this consists of reflex withdrawal, by contraction of flexor muscles, of a limb which is subjected to intense stimulation. This reflex is of course a common enough experience in association with painful or startling stimuli, but it is important to realize that it occurs (without its conscious sensory concomitant) in the isolated spinal cord. It is again homeostatic; not in the sense that it restores the organism (or part of it) to an original position in space, or an original state of muscle tension, but in that it restores the organism to equilibrium with respect to its external environment.

The mechanism of the withdrawal reflex, being primitive, is neurologically somewhat more complicated. It involves the convergence of a number of Aδ primary afferents from high-threshold receptors on neurones in the dorsal horn of the spinal grey matter. These neurones, in their turn, excite the ventral horn motoneurones innervating the appropriate flexor muscles. Thus it is a polysynaptic reflex, and probably involves convergence (spatial summation) at both synaptic levels. The primary afferent fibres involved in this reflex come not only from the tegument (skin and subjacent tissues), but also from high threshold receptors in the deep tissues, such as Group III muscle afferents. The central connections of these neurones are very profuse. Thus although in the intact animal the flexor reflex usually only involves the limb stimulated, in the spinal animal, with suitable intensities of stimulation, all flexor muscles may be brought into play, as may the detrusor muscles of the bladder, so that the animal curls up and micturates. This is known as the mass reflex. Under normal conditions, it must be assumed that tonic inhibitory control from higher centres serves to localize reflex withdrawal to muscles whose motoneurones are undergoing the most intensive afferent bombardment.

It should be noted that, in the presence of adequate stimuli, primitive withdrawal (flexion) reflexes will always predominate over extensor reflexes, which are normally brought into play by stimuli of lower energy. Therefore, in physiological terms, high

energy stimuli not only provoke flexion reflexes but inhibit extensor reflexes; it is conceivable that this latter may come about by
presynaptic inhibition of extensor reflex afferents by the smaller
flexor afferent fibres.

Under carefully controlled conditions of supraliminal stimulation, flexion of the stimulated limb is accompanied by extension
of the contralateral limb (crossed extensor reflex); this obviously
stabilizes the stance of the organism when the flexed limb is off

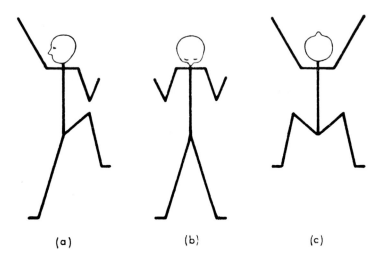

(a)   (b)   (c)

FIG. 20. Tonic neck reflexes (a) Rotation: face limbs extend,
occipital limbs flex. (b) Flexion: upper limbs flex, lower limbs
extend. (c) Extension: upper limbs extend, lower limbs flex.

the ground. There may even occur extension of the other (anterior
or posterior, as the case may be) ipsilateral limb and flexion of its
opposite number; this prepares the animal for movement away
from the offending stimulus.

TONIC NECK REFLEXES (FIG. 20)

These represent perhaps the most sophisticated level of integrated
activity intrinsic to the spinal cord. Primary afferent fibres coming
mainly from receptors in the joints by which the head moves on

the trunk, reach the spinal cord in the dorsal roots of the first two pairs of cervical nerves. Three kinds of responses are seen:

1. When the head is rotated, the limbs on the side to which the face is turned extend, while those on the 'occipital' side flex.

2. When the head is flexed at the neck (chin-to-chest position), the forelimbs flex and the hindlimbs extend.

3. When the head is extended on the trunk (stargazing position), the hindlimbs flex and the forelimbs extend.

It may be taken as an axiom of neurophysiology that no synapse exists only to transmit nervous messages in an unaltered form. Modification of information can and does occur at all synaptic junctions. Thus the intrinsic mechanisms of the spinal cord which have been described in this chapter are under constant control from higher centres; for example, the righting reflexes described above normally require facilitation from midbrain centres, and are only seen in the spinal animal when stimulant drugs are used. It must, however, be stressed that descending inhibitory effects are at least as important as facilitatory ones in modifying intrinsic spinal behaviour. Some of these control mechanisms will be described in subsequent chapters.

CHAPTER SEVEN

The Lower Brain Stem and Cranial Nerve Nuclei

Although the brain stem shows essentially the same basic morphology as the spinal cord, its structure becomes more and more complicated as we proceed rostrally, and so it is less easy to recognize the primitive pattern. But it must be remembered that the grey matter throughout the cord and brainstem forms a continuous core, whose brainstem part is called the **tegmentum**; and that many fibre tracts, both ascending and descending, can be traced throughout all these parts of the CNS. By remembering the essential continuity of both grey and white matter, it should be possible to develop and retain a holistic view of the structure of the brain stem, instead of committing to memory a series of discrete cross-sections, apparently unrelated to one another.

The part of the brain stem immediately adjoining the spinal cord is the **medulla oblongata**. Its caudalmost part closely resembles the cord in structure (Fig. 21). It differs chiefly in that the corticospinal tracts, instead of occupying the lateral white columns, lie on the ventral aspect of the brain stem (a position they occupy throughout). At the junction of medulla and cord, these fibre tracts pass from the ventral aspect of the medulla (where they form an elevation known as the **pyramids**) to the lateral column of the opposite side of the cord; this change in position is known as the **decussation of the pyramids**. Following the brain stem rostrally, this change in fibre architecture may be seen to have two effects on the structure of the brain stem:

1. Most caudally, where the fibres are actually streaming across (decussating) from one (ventral) pyramid to the opposite lateral column, the anterior median sulcus is obliterated, and the ventral horn of the grey matter is as it were cut off from access

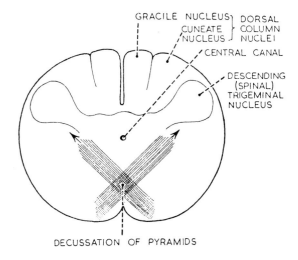

FIG. 21. Semidiagrammatic coronal section through the medulla oblongata at its junction with the spinal cord.

to the surface (Fig. 21), so that the orderly emergence of ventral roots is interrupted.

2. A little more rostrally, the position of the pyramids on the ventral surface of the medulla causes the central core of grey matter to occupy a *relatively* more dorsal position than it does in the spinal cord, so that the central canal now appears to be a good deal nearer the dorsal than the ventral aspect of the medulla.

Only a small distance rostral to the decussation of the pyramids the white fibres of the dorsal (posterior) columns terminate in cell masses (nuclei) which lie in direct continuity with the fibres (Fig. 21). These are known as the **gracile** (medial) and **cuneate** (lateral) nuclei, or more simply and functionally, as the **dorsal column nuclei.** They form small elevations or tubercles on the dorsal aspect of the medulla. Secondary sensory fibres arise from these nuclei, eventually to pass rostrally as the **medial lemniscus.** But these fibres, before turning rostrally, pass ventrolaterally through the grey matter, under the central canal, to attain the opposite side of the brain stem in a position immediately dorsal to the pyramids. While crossing, these fibres of the medial lemniscus form one group of **internal arcuate fibres.**

The architectural effect of the ending of the dorsal white columns, while the secondary fibres arising from the dorsal column nuclei pass ventrolaterally under the central canal, is to bring the central canal right up on to the dorsal surface of the medulla, so that it opens out, the dorsal surface of the brain stem forming its floor. The roof is formed by the cerebellum, which overlies the brain stem at this point, and the whole widely dilated and displaced canal forms a cavity called the **fourth ventricle.**

Two other features mark the medulla, and explain its structural differentiation. Those (ascending) fibres of the dorsolateral white columns of the cord which do not belong to the (descending) corticospinal system diverge laterally along the margins of the fourth ventricle, and at the rostral limit of the medulla oblongata, they turn rather sharply dorsally into the cerebellum. Thus these fibres, which in the cord are known as the dorsal spinocerebellar tract, form the bulk of the caudalmost of three fibre bundles which on each side tether the cerebellum to the brain stem. This is known as the **inferior cerebellar peduncle** or **restiform body.**

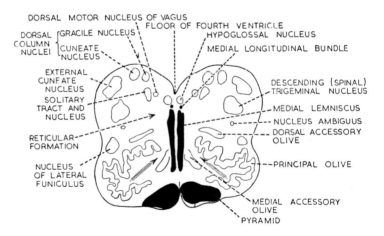

FIG. 22. Semidiagrammatic coronal section through the open (rostral) part of the medulla. This is the only level at which all six columns of sensory and motor cells are represented (see p. 13).

Also in the rostral part of the medulla is found, lying dorso-lateral to the pyramid, an elevation known as the **olive** (Fig. 22). On cross section this can be seen to be a purse-shaped mass of grey matter, the **inferior olivary nucleus**, open on its medial side. Separating the two olives from the midline are the fibres of the medial lemnisci. Fibres stream out of the open 'mouth' of the olive and cross laterodorsally through the medial lemniscus and grey matter to reach the inferior cerebellar peduncle of the opposite side. These olivo-cerebellar fibres therefore form a second (and slightly more rostrally placed) group of internal arcuate fibres.

Turning now to the central core of grey matter of the medulla oblongata (**tegmentum**), certain features can be seen to be direct continuations of the arrangement in the spinal cord. The large motor cells which form lamina IX of the ventral horn of the spinal grey matter lie ventrolateral to the central canal. In the medulla, this column of cells occupies the same position, but this means that in the rostral (open) part of the medulla, these cells will lie just below the floor of the fourth ventricle, close to the midline. These cells come to an end at the rostral limit of the medulla. Their efferent fibres form the twelfth cranial or hypoglossal nerve, which goes to innervate the muscles of the tongue; therefore the motoneurones in the medulla are known as the **hypoglossal nucleus** (Figs. 22 and 25) and the fibres emerge between the pyramid and the olive. Ventral to the hypoglossal nuclci, and above the medial lemniscus, lies the caudal end of the **medial longitudinal bundle** (fasciculus) (Fig. 22) (see p. 69 infra).

Those cells of the dorsal horn around which fibres fired by painful and thermal stimuli end, are continued up through the medulla as the **spinal (descending) nucleus of the trigeminal nerve** (Figs. 21 and 22). The nucleus therefore lies lateral, and slightly ventral, to the posterior white columns and their nuclei. In the upper part of the medulla it lies below the floor of the fourth ventricle, separated from it by certain special nuclei to be mentioned later. The spinal trigeminal nucleus receives fibres bringing impulses generated by painful and thermal stimuli from the face. These fibres lie between the nucleus and the periphery of the medulla, and are known as the **spinal tract of the trigeminal nerve** (Fig. 22).

Those cells in the medial part of lamina VI in the cord (Clarke's column) which give rise to the dorsal spinocerebellar tract are represented in the medulla by a group of cells which lie immediately beneath the floor of the fourth ventricle in its caudal part, immediately lateral to the dorsal column nuclei. It is rather confusingly known as the **lateral (external) cuneate nucleus** (Fig. 22), for it has no functional connection with the more lateral of the two dorsal column nuclei (**cuneate nucleus**). The lateral cuneate nucleus sends its fibres into the inferior cerebellar peduncle of the same side. It lies dorsal to the spinal trigeminal nucleus.

It will be recalled that between the first thoracic and second lumbar segments of the cord there are motor cells in the lateral part of the grey matter which give rise to autonomic motor fibres. If the spinal grey matter were rounded off, rather than butterfly-shaped, it would easily be seen that these cells would lie dorsolateral to the larger (somatic) motor cells in lamina IX of the ventral horn. In the medulla this column reappears as the **dorsal motor nucleus of the vagus** (Figs. 22 and 25). It lies dorsolateral to the hypoglossal nucleus under the floor of the fourth ventricle. It represents the cerebral autonomic outflow, and its fibres, which pass into the tenth cranial (vagus) nerve, leave the medulla dorsal to the olive.

Lateral to the dorsal motor nucleus of the vagus lies a sensory nucleus, unrepresented in the cord, known as the **nucleus of the solitary tract.** Sensory fibres of the tenth, ninth and seventh nerves, probably from special sense organs of taste, running in the **solitary tract,** which surrounds the nucleus, end in its rostral part (Figs. 22 and 25); some ascending fibres from the spinal cord terminate in its caudal part.

Somewhat ventral or ventrolateral to the spinal trigeminal nucleus, lies a narrow column of large motor cells. This is the **nucleus ambiguus** (Fig. 22). Its fibres, which pass out dorsal to the olive, go to innervate striated muscles which are derived from the branchial arch mesoderm (palate, pharynx, larynx). For this embryological reason, these cells have no homologue in the grey matter of the spinal cord.

Just as the gracile and cuneate nuclei are embedded in the dorsal columns and receive their fibres from them, so there is a nucleus embedded in the ascending anterolateral column at medullary level. The **nucleus of the lateral funiculus** (lateral reticular nucleus) lies dorsolateral to the olive (Fig. 22). It differs from the dorsal column nuclei in that it does not receive all the ascending fibres from the white column in which it is embedded—many of them pass on up to more rostral parts of the brain stem. The axons of cells in the nucleus of the lateral funiculus pass to the cerebellum in the inferior peduncle of the same side.

Most of the named specific nuclei which have been described in the preceding paragraphs lie on the periphery of the grey core of the medulla. The more central parts of the medullary grey matter are broken up into small groups by the decussating and interlacing internal arcuate fibres, and is therefore called the **reticular formation.** It represents an expanded part of lamina VII of the cord. Many ascending fibres from the anterolateral columns of the cord terminate in the reticular formation. Some groups of reticular cells have axons which project rostrally to higher levels of the brain stem, while others (reticulospinal neurones) have axons which pass down into the spinal cord in the anterior and lateral white columns

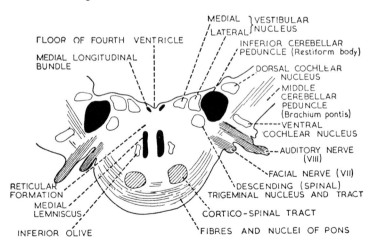

FIG. 23. Semidiagrammatic coronal section through the caudal (open) pons.

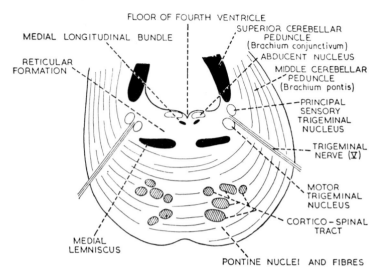

FIG. 24. Semidiagrammatic coronal section through the rostral pons.

(Fig. 16). Some reticular cells have been shown to possess dichotomizing axons of which one branch passes upwards and one downwards.

The portion of the brain stem lying rostral to the medulla oblongata is the **pons** (Figs. 23 and 24). It is characterized by very thick bundles of fibres which run transversely across its ventral aspect and turn up into the cerebellum—hence the analogy with a bridge.

Actually these fibres do not encircle the pons. They arise from grey matter in its ventral part, the **nuclei pontis.** These scattered nuclei receive descending axons which run with the corticospinal fibres, and give off laterally-running fibres which pass up into the cerebellum as the **middle peduncle (brachium pontis).** The middle peduncle is the largest and outermost of the cerebellar peduncles. Crossing the transverse pontine fibres at right angles, and broken up by them into small bundles, are the descending corticospinal fibres.

Above this basal part of the pons, and below the floor of the fourth ventricle, which attains its greatest width just caudal to the middle peduncle, lie the central grey matter and the long ascending white tracts. In the medulla, the medial lemnisci lie between the olives, and look in cross section like two books standing up. In the pons the olive is no longer present, and the books have fallen outwards, i.e. the medial lemniscus is now lying transversely, just above the pontine nuclei and fibres, instead of vertically. Thus the lateral end of the medial lemniscus comes to be mingled with the long ascending fibres from the anterolateral quadrant of the cord, which are now no longer separated from it by the olive.

Continuing rostrally from the spinal trigeminal nucleus is the **principal sensory trigeminal nucleus** (Fig. 24). This differs in cell structure from the spinal nucleus. Ventromedial to this is the **motor trigeminal nucleus**, whose efferent fibres go to innervate the muscles of mastication. Being branchiomotor in origin and function, this nucleus is in line with the nucleus ambiguus. The fibres of the fifth (trigeminal) nerve enter and leave the brain stem at mid-pontine level. At the rostral end of the medulla, still in line with (but discrete from) the motor trigeminal nucleus and the nucleus ambiguus is another branchiomotor nucleus—the **facial (seventh nerve) nucleus.**

Special sensory nuclei concerned with the vestibular and cochlear divisions of the eighth cranial nerve lie on the dorsal surface of the brain stem at the medullo-pontine junction. The auditory nerve enters the brain stem on the under surface of the inferior cerebellar peduncle (restiform body). At its point of entry lies a groups of cells known as the **ventral cochlear nucleus,** around which some bifurcating fibres of the cochlear division terminate (Fig. 23). The **dorsal cochlear nucleus,** which is more intricately organized, lies a little further rostrally, on the rostro-dorsal extremity of the restiform body, just rostro-lateral to the lateral extremity (lateral angle) of the fourth ventricle. The other branches of the cochlear division end in this nucleus. Secondary fibres from the cochlear nuclei pass inwards towards the central grey matter as the **trapezoid body.** Some of these fibres relay further in certain scattered nuclei of this region, known as **trapezoid nuclei** and **superior olive.** Both direct and indirect fibres turn rostrally as the **lateral lemniscus,** the auditory pathway which in the upper pons lies laterodorsal to the medial lemniscus.

The **vestibular nuclei** (Fig. 25), in which the vestibular division of the eighth nerve terminates, lie medial to the dorsal cochlear nucleus, in the lateralmost part of the floor of the fourth ventricle, dorsal to the sensory trigeminal nuclei, and lateral to the rostral end of nucleus of the solitary tract. The vestibular nuclei form a complex group in which four divisions are usually recognized. Of these, the **lateral vestibular nucleus** contains

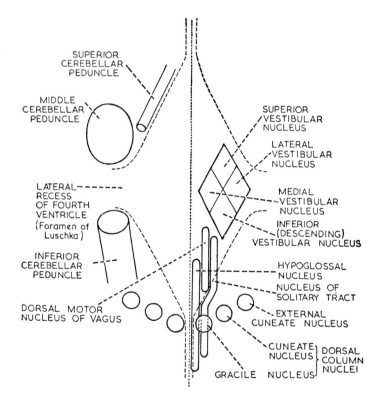

FIG. 25. Dorsal projection of the floor of the fourth ventricle. Structures located in the floor are shown on the right; the cerebellar peduncles, forming the lateral boundaries of the ventricle, are shown on the left.

giant motor cells whose axons pass down into the anterior funiculus of the cord as the **vestibulospinal tract.** The other vestibular nuclei are connected with the motor nuclei of the extraocular muscles in the somatic efferent column and the dorsal motor nucleus of the vagus by means of the **medial longitudinal bundle** (fasciculus) (Figs. 22, 23, 24, 26 and 27).

The fourth ventricle narrows rostrally, due to the approximation of the **superior cerebellar peduncles** (Fig. 24) which form its lateral boundary. These fibre columns are the smallest and most medially placed of the cerebellar peduncles. As the superior peduncle (brachium conjunctivum) approaches its fellow of the opposite side, the space between the two is roofed in by an ependymal membrane, the **superior medullary velum.** The ventricle thus narrows to a passage, known as the **cerebral aqueduct** (of Sylvius). The aqueduct is the representative of the central canal in the midbrain (mesencephalon), and in this region a plate of grey matter, the **tectum** (roof) lies above the aqueduct.

The **tectum** is differentiated into four rounded elevations, the **corpora quadrigemina.** The rostral pair is known as the

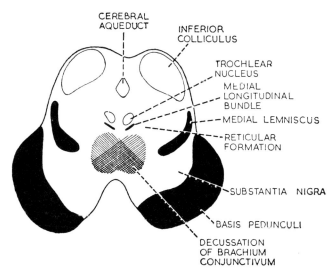

FIG. 26. Semidiagrammatic coronal section through the caudal midbrain, at the level of the inferior colliculi.

superior colliculi (Fig. 27), and the caudal as the **inferior colliculi** (Fig. 26). Many fibres of the lateral (auditory) lemniscus end in the inferior colliculus, while the superior colliculus receives fibres from the optic pathway (q.v.). Both pairs of colliculi, but chiefly the superior, receive fibres from, and transmit fibres to, the cervical spinal cord, in the anterior funiculi (spinotectal and tectospinal tracts). These tracts subserve reflex head turning in response to visual and auditory stimuli respectively.

Beneath the floor of the aqueduct on either side of the midline, lie three more somatic efferent cranial nerve nuclei, all concerned with the innervation of the extrinsic muscles of the eyeball. The

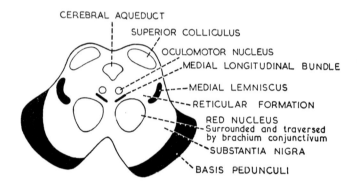

CEREBRAL AQUEDUCT
SUPERIOR COLLICULUS
OCULOMOTOR NUCLEUS
MEDIAL LONGITUDINAL BUNDLE
MEDIAL LEMNISCUS
RETICULAR FORMATION
RED NUCLEUS
Surrounded and traversed by brachium conjunctivum
SUBSTANTIA NIGRA
BASIS PEDUNCULI

FIG. 27. Semidiagrammatic coronal section through the rostral midbrain, at the level of the superior colliculi.

most caudal of these, the **abducent** (sixth nerve) **nucleus,** lies in the floor of the rostral part of the fourth ventricle; so that properly speaking it is situated in the pons (Fig. 24). The abducent nucleus is encircled medially, dorsally, and laterally by the efferent fibres of the facial nucleus, producing an elevation in the floor of the fourth ventricle known as the **facial colliculus.** In the midbrain proper, bounding the aqueduct ventrolaterally, lie the **oculomotor** and **trochlear nuclei** (third and fourth cranial nerves) (Figs. 26 and 27). Below these nuclei, in the midbrain tegmentum is the mesencephalic reticular substance. The peasized **red nucleus** can be seen within it, with the naked eye (Fig. 27). The reason for the clear delineation of the red nucleus is that it is en-sheathed by the fibres of the brachium conjunctivum (superior cerebellar peduncle), which have decussated on entering the midbrain.

Whereas in the pons the long descending tracts (corticospinal and frontopontine) extend lateromedially across the brainstem, in the midbrain they are collected on the lateral side of the ventral aspect of the brainstem, with increasing divergence between the **cerebral peduncles** of the two sides as they are traced rostrally (Fig. 27). This is because they are to become continuous with the white matter of the widely separated cerebral hemispheres.

The fibre tracts are contained in the ventralmost part of cerebral peduncle, known as the **basis pedunculi.** Its dorsal part merges with the central tegmentum, and contains some conspicuously dark, melanin-pigmented, grey matter called the **substantia nigra.** The substantia nigra, together with the more dorsally placed red nucleus, forms a part of the so-called **extrapyramidal motor system** (vide infra).

Intrinsic Brainstem Mechanisms

Under normal circumstances, the brainstem, like the spinal cord, is of course under the domination of higher levels of the neuraxis, by means of afferent fibres from higher centres. However, when it is released from higher control by transection in a coronal plane between the superior and inferior colliculi (classical decerebration), certain intrinsic mechanisms can be studied. It should be noted that the plane of intercollicular decerebration passes caudal to upper midbrain structures, including the red nucleus and sub-stantia nigra. On the other hand the cerebellum remains attached to the brainstem, and its connections through the inferior peduncle and the descending limb of the brachium conjunctivum (pp. 62 and 69) are intact. Cerebellar influences will not be considered in this chapter.

DECEREBRATE RIGIDITY

The most striking result of decerebration (in the cat) is the immediate production of extreme hypertonicity in the extensor muscles of the limbs and of the neck, so that the animal stands like a statue and can as easily be knocked over.

Two structures, when released from inhibition by higher centres, contribute to the maintenance of decerebrate rigidity. These are (a) the rostral and lateral parts of the **reticular formation** of the lower brain stem, and (b) the **vestibular nuclei.** Under these headings we shall deal, in the present chapter, both with their role in decerebrate rigidity and with some of their other functional properties.

The Reticular Formation

The rostral and lateral part of the reticular formation of the isolated brainstem exhibits spontaneous neuronal activity, and is a **facilitatory region.** Descending effects from this region are principally exerted on extensor γ-motoneurones, and so contribute to the maintenance of extensor rigidity mainly by facilitation of the stretch reflex (γ-loop). It follows, therefore, that dorsal root section, by interrupting the afferent arc of the stretch reflex, largely abolishes the reticulospinal component of decerebrate rigidity.

The more caudal and ventromedial part of the reticular formation is normally electrically silent, i.e. it does not show spontaneous activity in the decerebrate preparation. Stimulation experiments show that this region is an **inhibitory centre,** in that it is able, through the intermediary of spinal interneurones, to bring about inhibition of both motoneurones and interneurones concerned with upward transmission of information.

Within the general facilitatory and inhibitory regions of the medullary reticular formation at the level of the vagal nucleus are to be found the **inspiratory** and **expiratory** parts respectively of the so-called **respiratory centre.** Rhythmic discharges from the inspiratory centre bring about contraction of the diaphragm and intercostal muscles; this would occur at an intrinsic and invariable rate in the absence of afferent signals. Normally, however, afferent impulses travelling in the vagus nerve from pulmonary stretch receptors and CO_2-sensitive chemoreceptors in the carotid sinus influence both the inhibitory expiratory centre and the facilitatory inspiratory centre and so bring about variations in the depth and rate of respiration which are exquisitely adjusted to the requirement of the organism.

In these same vago-reticular regions are less well-defined 'centres' for the control of blood pressure and cardiac activity. Unlike the lungs, the heart beats through its own intrinsic rhythmicity, so there are no systolic and diastolic centres corresponding to the inspiratory and expiratory centres. But cardiac activity is influenced through the vagus nerve, in response to afferent information arriving in the medulla oblongata from baroreceptors in the carotid body. Due to the overlapping distribution of these areas within the reticular formation, respiratory and cardiac volume and rate as well as blood pressure variations are mutually interdependent.

The Vestibular Nuclei
Destruction of the vestibular nuclei largely abolishes decerebrate rigidity. The strongly facilitatory effect on extensor motoneurones is mediated by the vestibulospinal pathway arising in the lateral vestibular nucleus. Unlike the reticular component, the vestibular component is not significantly affected by dorsal root section, showing that the facilitation is therefore principally exerted on α-motoneurones. Vestibulospinal activity in the decerebrate state is itself due to tonic input from the vestibular apparatus (sacculus), destruction of which (or section of the vestibular portion of the eighth nerve) therefore also abolishes the vestibular component of decerebrate rigidity. This functional connection is not surprising when it is recalled that the extensor muscles involved are in fact antigravity muscles.

Vestibular reflexes come into play during free fall. Vestibular reflexes first correct the position of the head and body with respect to gravity, and then cause the limbs to extend. The result is that 'pussy-cat always lands on her feet'.

The interconnection of vestibular and oculomotor nuclei (III,

IV, and VI) through the medial longitudinal bundle enable the eyes to remain smoothly fixated upon an object while the head is moving; this constitutes the **vestibulo-ocular reflexes**. Due to the viscosity (and hence inertia) of the fluid in the semicircular canals, rapid and irregular changes in head position result in a failure to synchronize head and eye movements, and because of the connections of the medial longitudinal bundle with the vagal nucleus and adjacent reticular formation, nausea and sometimes vomiting (motion sickness) are produced. Damage to the vestibular apparatus, nerve, or nuclei causes failure to maintain peripheral ocular fixation, so that the eyes wander slowly back to a central position, corrected by rapid jerks towards the affected side; this is known as **nystagmus**.

CHAPTER EIGHT

The Diencephalon

The diencephalon is the rostralmost part of the brain stem, and is embedded between the cerebral hemispheres. Between the mesencephalon and diencephalon, the brain stem bends forwards (ventrally) at almost a right angle (Fig. 28), which makes it rather difficult in sections to follow the continuity of white and grey structures.

In order to see the diencephalon from above, it would be necessary to remove the upper (dorsal) parts of the cerebral hemispheres and the **corpus callosum** joining them. The most obvious structures in the diencephalon then are the two **thalami**, separated by the cavity of the **third ventricle**, though frequently joined across it by a variable-sized glial **interthalamic connexus**. Each

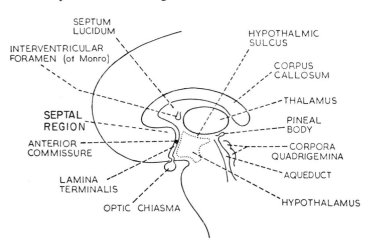

FIG. 28. Median sagittal section, to show the mesodiencephalic junction, the corpus callosum, and the structures in the wall of the third ventricle.

75

thalamus, seen from above, is egg-shaped (Fig. 29) with its little end pointing forward and the two medial borders parallel to one another. The big (posterior, caudal) ends are fairly widely divergent, and embrace the rostralmost part of the mesencephalic tectum. Looked at in side view, it would be seen that the caudal end (**pulvinar**) of the thalamus forms a backward projection beneath whose overhang lie two rounded projections, the **medial** and **lateral geniculate bodies**. The medial geniculate body can be seen quite clearly to be connected to the inferior colliculus by

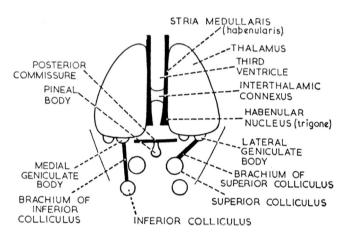

FIG. 29. Diagrammatic view of the diencephalon and midbrain from above.

a band of fibres known as the **brachium of the inferior colliculus**. The lateral geniculate body on the other hand receives the **optic tract**, which can be seen winding round the midbrain to reach it.

The thalamus is continuous with part of the grey matter of the mesencephalic tegmentum. All secondary sensory neurones, as well as the efferent outflow from the cerebellum (brachium conjunctivum) end in it. Thus it receives the optic tract (in the lateral geniculate body), the auditory pathway, via the inferior colliculus and its brachium (in the medial geniculate body), the medial lemniscus and the spinothalamic tract, in addition to many fibres proceeding rostrally from the reticular formation of the lower brain stem (see Chapters 11 and 12).

The long descending tracts, which in the midbrain occupy the cerebral peduncle (basis pedunculi), lie below and lateral to the tegmental grey matter. As they are traced antidromically up into the cerebral hemispheres, they are seen to lie on the lateral side of the thalamus, where they are segregated into a well-marked band of white matter known as the **internal capsule** (see Chapter 9). To attain this position, the white matter of the basis pedunculi has obviously moved dorsolaterally relative to the grey matter.

Viewed from within the cavity of the third ventricle (Fig. 28) the thalamus forms the dorsal part of its lateral wall, and is bounded ventrally by a groove, the **hypothalamic sulcus**. The ventral part of the wall of the third ventricle below this groove consists of the grey matter of the **hypothalamus**. The hypo-thalamus is the diencephalic centre of the autonomic nervous system. From the more rostral part of the floor of the third ventricle a funnel-shaped depression, the **infundibulum**, leads to the stalk of the pituitary gland. Thus this important endocrine organ, and particularly its posterior portion (pars nervosa) is in direct continuity with the hypothalamus.

The third ventricle and diencephalon are bounded rostrally by a membrane, the **lamina terminalis**, which passes down from the rostral tip of the corpus callosum above to the optic chiasma below (Fig. 28). Embedded in it is the **anterior commissure**, which passes transversely across the rostral boundary of the ventricle (Fig. 28). In the lateral wall, behind the lamina terminalis lies the **anterior column of the fornix**, a thick band of white fibres passing down into the **mammillary body** in the floor of the posterior part of the hypothalamus. Between the anterior column of the fornix and the rostral pole of the thalamus is a hole leading into the **lateral ventricle**: this is the **interventricular foramen** (of Monro) (Fig. 28).

The dorsolateral boundary of the third ventricle is formed by a ridge of white matter which passes from the front of the ventricle along the dorsomedial border of the thalamus to end in a small lump of grey matter attached to the medial aspect of the pulvinar. The fibre tract is called the **striae medullaris** (habenularis), and leads to the **habenular nuclei** or trigone (Fig. 29). Springing from the region of the habenular trigone on each side is the stalk of the **pineal gland,** which is therefore a small (but rather variable-sized) midline structure at the caudo-dorsal extremity of the third ventricle. Rostral to this point the roof of the ventricle is formed by the **tela choroidea** of the third ventricle, which passes between (above) the striae medullaris of the two sides.

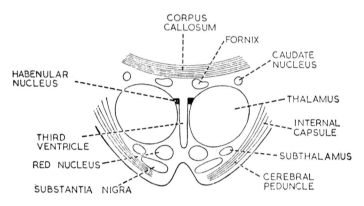

FIG. 30. Semidiagrammatic coronal section through the mesodiencephalic junction. Compare with Figs. 27 and 28.

Behind and below the habenular trigones and pineal stalk lies the **posterior commissure** (Fig. 29). This is a double fibre bundle which forms the posterior (caudal) boundary of the third ventricle; caudal to this point the ventricle narrows into the aqueduct of the midbrain.

If the meso-diencephalic junction is viewed in coronal section (Fig. 30), a small cigar-shaped mass of grey matter will be seen below the lateral part of the thalamus, separated from it by white fibres. This is the **subthalamus,** an important but ill-understood motor centre belonging to the extrapyramidal motor system (Chapter 13).

CHAPTER NINE

The Telencephalon

The **telencephalon** or forebrain consists of the two **cerebral hemispheres**, which in man are so large as to hide the diencephalon and midbrain. The two hemispheres are separated by the **median longitudinal fissure**, when viewed from above. At the bottom of this fissure may be seen a very extensive band of transversely running white fibres, which form a commissure connecting the two hemispheres. This is the **corpus callosum** (Figs. 28 and 30), whose fibres (numbering 10×10^6) interconnect mirror-image points in the two hemispheres. If the corpus callosum be split longitudinally, the third ventricle, and therefore the diencephalon, can be seen below it.

While the dissector must of necessity start from the external surface of the forebrain, the continuity of this description will be better served by describing first those parts of the telencephalon which border on the diencephalon, which is, as it were, invaginated into the forebrain.

The diencephalo–telencephalic junction can best be understood by the simultaneous study of coronal and horizontal sections in which the third and lateral ventricles and their relations are included. The third ventricle is the cavity of the diencephalon (see Chapter 8) and all the structures bounding it belong to the diencephalon. Each lateral ventricle is the cavity of the corresponding (telencephalic) hemisphere, although it is related medially to the thalamus, which is a diencephalic nucleus; all other structures related to the lateral ventricles belong to the forebrain. To understand the anatomy of the lateral ventricle and its relations is to understand the anatomy of the interior of the cerebral hemispheres. The whole of the forebrain grows in a semi-helical fashion (Fig. 31), starting from a transverse axis running through

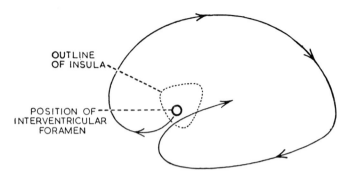

FIG. 31. Diagram to show the semi-helical fashion in which the forebrain grows, starting from a transverse axis through the interventricular foramen.

the interventricular foramen (Figs. 28 and 31). Because of this, the lateral ventricles and structures contained within the forebrain are mostly C-shaped.

Seen in side view (Fig. 32), the lateral ventricle is like a drawn-out letter C with a postero-superior prolongation, called the **posterior horn.** The part just in front of the posterior horn is the **body,** while the extreme rostral end is called the **anterior horn.** The lower curved part is the **inferior horn;** this meets the body and posterior horn at the **collateral trigone.** The interventricular

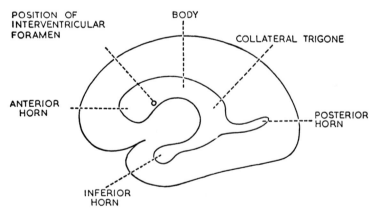

FIG. 32. Outline of the lateral ventricle projected on to a lateral view of the cerebral hemisphere.

foramen (Fig. 28) by which the lateral ventricle communicates with the third ventricle, lies at the junction between the body and the anterior horn.

Ignoring for the moment the posterior horn, the C-shape of the main part of the lateral ventricle is impressed upon it by the **caudate nucleus,** one of the deep grey masses of the telencephalon, which it follows. The caudate nucleus (Fig. 33) has a large globular **head** and a thin attenuated **body** and **tail.** The head lies in front of the thalamus, while the body and tail are wrapped around its outer edge. Thus the head and body of the nucleus lie

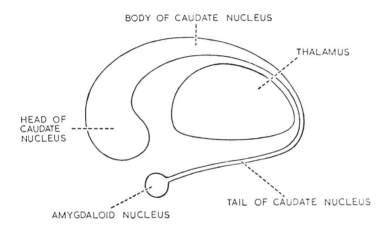

FIG. 33. Diagram to show the relationship of the caudate and amygdaloid nuclei to the thalamus.

in the floor of the anterior horn and body of the lateral ventricle; anterior to the collateral trigone lies the junction of body and tail as they curve round the postero-external aspect of the thalamus; while the tail of the caudate nucleus forms the roof of the inferior horn of the ventricle.

Another C-shaped structure is intimately related to the lateral ventricle; this is the **hippocampus** and its rostral continuation the **fornix** (Fig. 34). The hippocampus is a cylindrical grey mass which lies in the floor of the inferior horn, and ends at the level of the collateral trigone. The fornix continues forwards over the dorsal aspect of the thalamus, but lies medial to the body of the caudate nucleus, not above it—in other words, while the C-shaped caudate nucleus may be said to be clamped vertically round the thalamus near its external border, the hippocampus-fornix complex lies eccentrically round the thalamus in such a way that the hippocampus lies under the lateral aspect of the thalamus (the tail of the caudate intervening) and the fornix lies over the medial aspect of the thalamus. At the rostro-medial end of the thalamus (Fig. 34), the fornix bends ventrally and slightly laterally, to

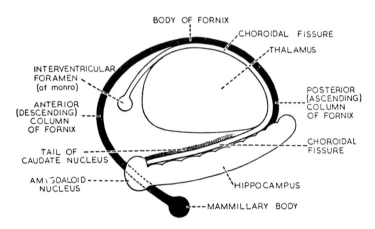

FIG. 34. Diagram to show the relationship of the hippocampus and fornix to the thalamus, and the choroidal fissure of the lateral ventricle.

become the anterior (descending) column of the fornix; it eventually goes to join the mammillary nuclei (bodies) in the caudal part of the floor of the third ventricle (hypothalamus). A space is left between the rostral pole of the thalamus and the anterior column of the fornix, and this allows the lateral ventricle to communicate with the third; it is known as the **interventricular foramen** (of Monro).

The pial **tela choroidea** is invaginated into the ventricle between the hippocampus and fornix on the one hand, and the thalamus on the other (Fig. 35). In its free edge lies the **choroid plexus** of the lateral ventricle. The choroid plexus itself becomes

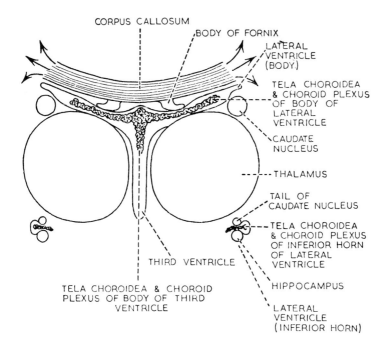

FIG. 35. Diagrammatic coronal section to show the choroidal fissures of the body and inferior horn of the lateral ventricle, and the corpus callosum. Compare Fig. 34.

continuous with the choroid plexus of the third ventricle through the interventricular foramen.

At the tip of the inferior horn of the lateral ventricle, both tail of caudate and hippocampus fuse into a globular grey mass known as the **amygdaloid nucleus** (Figs. 33 and 34), thus closing off the cavity of the ventricle. Note that owing to the shape of the caudate nucleus, the amygdaloid nucleus comes to lie under (ventral to) its head (Fig. 33).

The roof of the anterior horn and body of the lateral ventricle is formed by the transversely running fibres of the corpus callosum; the medial wall by the **septum pellucidum** (septum lucidum) which stretches between the under surface of the corpus callosum and the upper surface of the fornix (Fig. 28).

The corpus callosum itself, when cut through sagittally in the midline (Fig. 28) is seen to have the shape of an elongated hook. The point of the hook is the **rostrum**, and its bend the **genu**. Behind this lies the main part of the corpus callosum, the **body**, and it terminates caudally in a knob, the **splenium**. Now the corpus callosum lies more or less in the middle of the cerebral hemisphere and its fibres fan out to connect identical points in the cortex of both hemispheres. Thus if viewed in coronal section (Figs. 30 and 35), the fibres of the corpus callosum can be seen to turn upwards and downwards as well as running transversely outwards. Similarly in horizontal section its fibres can be seen running forwards and backwards from the rostral and caudal ends respectively, as well as transversely from the body. Because its rostral end (genu) is relatively nearer the frontal pole of the hemisphere than is its caudal end (splenium) to the occipital pole, the fibres fanning forward from the genu form a small pincer, the **forceps minor** while those fanning back from the splenium form a larger pincer, the **forceps major**. The forceps major will be seen to form the medial wall of the posterior horn of the lateral ventricle. Its lateral wall is formed by the **optic radiation**, a band of fibres running from the lateral geniculate body of the thalamus to the cortex on the medial aspect of the occipital pole of the hemisphere. The posterior horn is very variable in size, and is not infrequently completely lacking. The fibres of the corpus callosum interdigitate with the fibres going to and coming from the cortex from and to subcortical structures; this interdigitation of fibres in the white matter (centrum semi-ovale) of the hemisphere is known as the **corona radiata.**

The rostrum of the corpus callosum is joined to the optic chiasma by a membrane, the **lamina terminalis** (Fig. 28). We have already met this structure in the previous chapter, and it will be recognized as the anterior wall of the third ventricle and therefore the rostral boundary of the diencephalon. Embedded in the lamina terminalis is another commissural bundle, the **anterior commissure**, which joins the two temporal poles. Just behind the lamina terminalis is the anterior (descending) column of the fornix.

The fornices of the two sides start well apart, on the dorsal aspect of the hippocampi of the two hemispheres. After leaving the hippocampus at the collateral trigone, the fornices of the two sides bend forwards and medially, approaching one another; this caudal part of the fornix is known as the **posterior (ascending) column**. Dorsal to the thalamus, the fornices of the two sides run forward together as the **body of the fornix** (Figs. 30 and 35). At the point where they meet, some fibres run transversely from one fornix to the other. This is known as the **psalterium** or **hippocampal commissure**. The body of the fornix lies immediately beneath the body of the corpus callosum; but at the rostral pole of the thalamus, the body of the corpus callosum continues forward for some little distance, while the two fornices separate again turning downwards, outwards and eventually backwards as the descending (anterior) columns. It is the beginning of the anterior column which is attached to the under surface of the corpus callosum by the septum pellucidum. Between the septa of the two sides is a small space, the **cavum septi pellucidi**

The relations of the lateral ventricles are summarized in the table on the next page.

The caudate nucleus is not the only large grey mass in the depth of the cerebral hemisphere. Ventrolateral to its head lies the **lentiform nucleus,** which has the shape of a short cone, with its slightly convex base lying parallel with the lateral surface of the hemisphere (Fig. 36). The lentiform nucleus can be seen to be divided into three parts. Its outer segment is relatively dark in colour, and is known as the **putamen**. At its infero-medio-rostral corner the putamen is continuous with the ventrolateral corner of the head of the caudate nucleus (Fig. 36b). The two inner divisions of the lentiform nucleus are paler in colour, and are known together as the **globus pallidus**. At its caudal extremity, the globus pallidus is continuous with the substantia nigra of the midbrain; this continuity should remind us that the globus pallidus is in fact partly a diencephalic structure. On the outer surface of the lentiform nucleus, between it and the cortex, is a thin shield of grey matter known as the **claustrum**. Above the level of junction of the putamen and the head of the caudate

Relations of the Lateral Ventricles

	Ant. horn	Body	Inf. horn	Post. horn
Roof	Corpus callosum	Corpus callosum	Tail of caudate nucleus	Corpus callosum
Floor	Head of caudate nucleus	Thalamus and body of caudate nucleus	Hippocampus	
Medial wall	Septum pellucidum	Thalamus and fornix	Tela choroidea	Forceps major of corpus callosum
Lateral wall	Head of caudate nucleus	Body of caudate nucleus	Tail of caudate nucleus	Optic radiation

nucleus, fibre bundles can be seen with the naked eye passing between these two grey masses. For this reason, the lentiform and caudate nuclei are called the **corpus striatum**. The corpus striatum together with the claustrum and amygdaloid nucleus are known collectively as the **basal ganglia**.

Inspection of a horizontal section at the level of the middle of the head of the caudate nucleus (Fig. 36*a*) shows that there is a V-shaped interval filled with white fibres, and open laterally, between the lentiform nucleus laterally, and the head of the

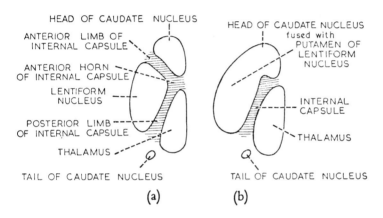

Fig. 36. Two diagrammatic horizontal sections to show the relationship between the thalamus, basal ganglia, and the internal capsule. (a) is at a more dorsal level than (b).

caudate nucleus antero-medially, with the thalamus lying postero-medial. This rather narrow passage, through which pass all the fibres going from the cortex to sub-telencephalic destinations (as well as many fibres passing up towards the cortex from lower centres) is known as the **internal capsule**. The segment between the caudate and the lentiform nuclei is the **anterior limb**, the apex of the V is the **genu**, and the part between the thalamus and lentiform nucleus, the **posterior limb**. The descending fibres of the internal capsule will eventually be assembled in the basis pedunculi of the midbrain, and it is important to be able to trace them down through the capsule to this level.

Examination of a horizontal section at a lower level (Fig. 36b) cutting through the lower part of the corpus striatum, shows that the putamen and the head of the caudate nucleus are fused together, so that the whole of the internal capsule is forced into the space previously occupied only by the posterior limb. This is made possible because most of the fibres in the posterior limb at the higher level are running from the thalamus to the cortex; thus they are not present at more ventral levels, allowing the fibres previously occupying the anterior limb to move into the posterior limb. Note therefore that the corticifugal fibres of the internal capsule are directed not only downwards but also to some extent backwards.

The ventralmost part of the internal capsule occupying the space between the lentiform nucleus and the thalamus, becomes directly continuous with the basis pedunculi. This will be understood if it is remembered that the midbrain joins the diencephalon and telencephalon at an angle; Fig. 37 shows the lowest horizontal section of the forebrain superimposed upon the slant-wise-cut transverse section of the midbrain (i.e. both sections in the same

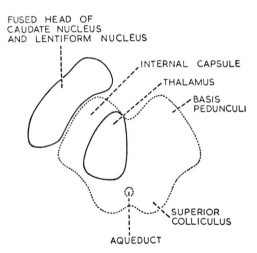

FIG. 37. Diagram of a horizontal section at the level of Fig. 36b superimposed on a coronal section of the midbrain (dotted outline), to show the manner in which the internal capsule becomes the basis pedunculi.

geometrical plane) which in fact lies immediately below it. It should also be remembered that as the fibres of the internal capsule are passing along the neuraxis, the picture to be borne in mind is not so much the horizontal section (though this is necessary for detail), but the coronal one (Fig. 30).

Lastly, a general consideration should be given of the outer grey covering of the forebrain, the **cerebral cortex**. The cortex varies in thickness from about $1\frac{1}{2}$mm (at the frontal pole) to $4\frac{1}{2}$mm (around the central sulcus, q.v.); the most recent estimates indicate that it contains some $2 \cdot 6 \times 10^9$ neurones. Because the surface area of the cortex (2–$2\frac{1}{2} \times 10^5$ sq mm) is much greater than that of the inner surface of its containing cranium, it is thrown into a series of ridges and furrows, called **gyri** and **sulci** respectively. About two-thirds of the cortex lies buried in the sulci.

Many of the sulci and gyri are completely haphazard in position and appearance, as are the pleats in a handkerchief bundled into the pocket. A small number, however, are constant, and these are the ones that the student should learn (Figs. 38 and 39).

Most of the constant sulci occupy the positions they do either because of the way the hemisphere grows, or because they have a functional significance; a small number of others are fairly constant, without having, so far as it is at present known, either of these excuses.

The sulci whose position is due to growth are marked in solid lines in Figs. 38 and 39. The fact that the forebrain grows in a semi-helical fashion (Fig. 31) is the cause of the appearance of the great **lateral fissure** (of Sylvius). The cortex at the point from which growth starts does not move, and so becomes covered by ontogenetically later cortex. This buried cortex is the **insula** (island of Reil) (Fig. 31). It has the shape of an inverted triangle, and is joined to the rest of the cortex by its (ventrally directed) apex, this being the **limen insulae**; elsewhere it is cut off by the **circular sulcus**. The pieces of cortex covering the insula are called the **opercula**—frontal, parietal and temporal, according to the bones under which they lie. The full extent and form of the insula can best be appreciated in horizontal and coronal sections. Note that the claustrum is co-extensive with the insula; and that

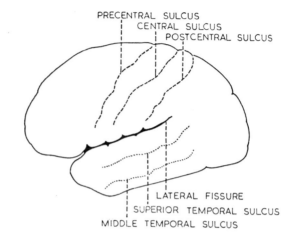

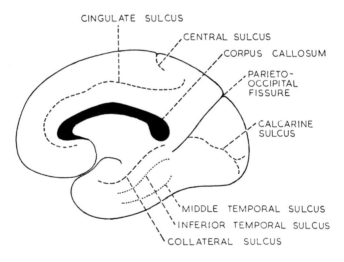

FIGS. 38 and 39. Lateral and infero-medial views of the cerebral hemisphere to show the constant sulci. Sulci which are constant owing to the manner in which the forebrain grows, but which have no functional significance, are shown as solid lines; sulci demarcating cortical zones of different function are shown as broken lines; other constant sulci, of no functional significance, are shown as dotted lines.

the 'axis of growth' passes medially from the centre of the insula to the interventricular foramen. The other sulcus due to growth is the **parieto-occipital fissure**, most of which is on the medial surface (Fig. 39) but whose apex usually cuts into the superolateral surface.

The sulci of functional significance (marked in broken lines on Figs. 38 and 39) may be subdivided into those marking or separating different functional areas of the cortex, and those separating different kinds of cortex from one another. Two main sulci belong to each group, those of the first being the **central** (Rolandic) and **calcarine** sulci. The central sulcus starts at the superomedial border of the hemisphere, behind its midpoint, and runs downwards and forwards over the superolateral surface, failing by a short distance to run into the lateral fissure. Parallel to the central sulcus, anterior and posterior to it respectively, are the **pre-** and **post-central** sulci. The two gyri thus demarcated are the **pre-** and **post-central** gyri. Cortical areas anterior to the central sulcus are motor in function, areas posterior to it are sensory.

On the medial surface of the hemisphere (Fig. 39) will be seen the deep calcarine sulcus, running from near the splenium of the corpus callosum to the occipital pole; the parieto-occipital fissure runs into its anterior end. The cortex on either side of the calcarine sulcus is the **visual area**, where sensory impulses originating in the optic nerves have their cortical termination.

Also on the medial surface, parallel to the corpus callosum, may be seen the **cingulate sulcus**. This separates the neocortex above it from the more primitive **allocortex**, here represented by the **cingulate gyrus**, lying between the sulcus of the same name and the corpus callosum.

On the inferior surface of the hemisphere (Fig. 39), the medial-most part of the cortex, next to the brain stem, is the **hippocampal gyrus** (not to be confused with the hippocampus). The hippocampal gyrus represents the phylogenetically oldest part of the cortex, and so is separated from the neocortical **fusiform gyrus** by the deep **collateral sulcus**, sometimes known as the occipitotemporal sulcus. Medially, the **hippocampal fissure** separates the hippocampal gyrus from the brain stem. The anterior end of the hippocampal gyrus is expanded into a club- or hook-shaped piece of cortex, which is known as the **uncus** (Fig. 39). The forward continuation of the collateral sulcus separating the uncus from the anterior end of the fusiform gyrus is called the **rhinal fissure**.

The cortical surface is arbitrarily divided by some of the sulci and fissures into four lobes, which are named after the bones of the cranial vault under which they lie. Thus the area in front of the central sulcus and above the lateral fissure is the **frontal lobe** (Fig. 38). An imaginary line is drawn down over the supero-lateral surface from the parieto-occipital fissure to the pre-occipital notch, an indentation in the latero-ventral border; behind this line lies the **occipital lobe**. The line of the lateral fissure is produced backwards to join this imaginary line, and the region below it is the **temporal lobe**. Behind the central sulcus, above the lateral fissure, and in front of the occipital lobe is the **parietal lobe**. The four lobes are used for convenience of nomenclature, but it should be noted that they do not correspond exactly to functional areas.

In the temporal lobe, below and parallel to the lateral fissure, are three constant sulci, the **superior, middle,** and **inferior temporal sulci**. Above each of these lies a gyrus of the same name. Below (medial to) the inferior temporal sulcus lies the fusiform gyrus.

The general structure of the neocortex will be considered in this chapter. There are essentially only two types of nerve cell in the cerebral cortex: a **pyramidal** cell and a **granular** cell, concerned with output and input functions respectively. The pyramidal cells have a long corticifugal axon, and an apical dendrite which goes up to the most superficial layer of the cortex. The granule cells are characterized by a profuse dendritic tree, while their axons are usually intracortical, and so may go off in any direction.

The neocortex is constructed in six layers. The outermost, or **molecular layer,** contains mostly the apical dendrites of the pyramidal cells, together with a small number of internuncial neurones. The innermost or **fusiform layer** contains internuncial and callosal neurones, whose axons end in the more superficial layers of their own or the opposite side. The intermediate layers are made up as a four-decker sandwich of granular and pyramidal cells. Layers II and IV are the **external** and **internal granular** layers respectively, while layers III and V are the **external** and **internal pyramidal layers**. The layers vary considerably in relative thickness in different areas of the cortex, as will be seen in the succeeding chapters.

CHAPTER TEN

Specific Sensory Systems

This chapter deals with the sensations that are appreciated in all parts of the body, and with the special senses of sight and hearing. Brief mention will be made here of the special senses of equilibration and taste, but the sense of smell will be reserved to the chapter on the Rhinencephalon.

Sensation must be dealt with before motor activity, for all movement is, in the final analysis a response to a sensory stimulus; the most profound of all paralyses is produced, not by cutting all the motor nerves, but by entirely blocking the sensory input to the CNS.

The four common cutaneous sensations—touch, pain, heat and cold, together with the deep sensations of pressure and kinaesthesia (sense of movement or position, from endings in and around joint capsules)—are referred to as the somatic sensations, since they can be felt in all parts of the body (soma), while the special senses require an elaborate end organ for their reception and transmutation into nervous energy. All the conscious sensations to be dealt with in this chapter have this in common: the appropriate stimuli generate impulses at the periphery which pass into the CNS, in which they pass by relay to the thalamus; thence by a final relay, the impulses pass to the appropriate part of the **cerebral cortex**.

When a peripheral receptor is adequately stimulated, impulses are transmitted to the central nervous system. Two mechanisms are capable of stopping this:

1. Adaptation in the receptor itself (see Chapter 5). Whether this process brings centripetal transmission to a halt or not depends entirely on whether the receptor is rapidly or slowly adapting.

2. Inhibition of transmission from receptor to primary afferent fibre by central action. To date, the only proven case of this mechanism in mammals is inhibition of transmission from cochlear hair cells to acoustic nerve axons by the efferent fibres of the olivo-cochlear bundle.

However, even when impulses have been set up in primary afferent fibres, they are not necessarily transmitted across the first central synapse to secondary neurones. Collaterals from other primary afferent fibres may prevent transmission by the mechanism of presynaptic inhibition. For example, the transmission of signals from Group I primary afferent fibres, arising from slowly-adapting muscle spindle receptors, may be presynaptically inhibited by impulses simultaneously arriving in high threshold cutaneous and muscular afferents.

It should be noted that only a suitably pre-activated centrifugal inhibitory system (as in (2) above) could conceivably prevent **any** afferent message coming from the periphery. By definition, receptor adaptation is bound to let the first impulse or impulses through. In the case of presynaptic inhibition quoted above, the greater conduction velocity in the Group I afferent ensures that the first impulses will get through before the more slowly conducted messages in higher threshold fibres (if activated simultaneously at the periphery) are able to inhibit transmission at the axon terminal.

Assuming the message from the periphery to have been transmitted safely across the first central synapse, the question then arises as to whether it will or will not cause an action potential to be generated in the secondary neurone. This depends on a number of factors, among which the following should be noted:

Convergence—in the primitive central nervous system, large numbers of peripheral axons, often of different specific modalities, converge onto one and the same central neurone. This condition is to a very large extent retained by higher vertebrates, although the development of larger numbers of central neurones allows the ratio to be lessened. It is easiest to deal first with the most highly evolved systems, among which the visual mechanism holds pride of place.

In the human retina there are somewhat over 100,000,000 photosensitive elements (rods and cones); but only about 1,000,000 fibres leave the eye in the optic nerve, as centripetal axons of the ganglion cells. Between the ganglion cells and the photoreceptors is a layer of bipolar cells, whose total number is somewhere between the two figures given above. From the most highly evolved part of the retina, the fovea, the ratio cones: bipolar cells: ganglion cells is known to be 1:1:1. This means that from the rest of the retina, there must be a convergence of rod and cone processes on to the peripheral bipolar cell processes, and a further convergence of central bipolar cell processes on to ganglion cells, such that the final ratio of receptors to ganglion cells is well over 100:1.

If we were to assume, for the purposes of the argument, that all retinal ganglion cells are at the same resting potential, and that they all require the same amount of transmitted afferent energy to cause them to fire, it could be said that the ganglion cells related to foveal cones (1:1) would be activated by 100 successive impulses originating in one receptor (temporal summation); while the ganglion cells related 100:1 to peripheral photoreceptors would be activated by 100 almost simultaneous impulses from different receptors (spatial summation).

Some other receptors, notably the cochlear hair cells and Pacinian corpuscles, like foveal cones, have a 1:1 ratio with primary afferent fibres. Most other receptors, however, converge on to primary afferent fibres (i.e. the peripheral end of the fibre branches to 'supply' several receptors). There is then further convergence of a number of primary afferent fibres onto central relay cells. The most sophisticated form of such convergence is unimodal, where only fibres carrying information from the same type of receptor (with, therefore, the same modality of selective sensitivity) converge on to relay cells. Such a situation exists, of course, in those retinal bipolar cells which converge onto ganglion cells, as well as in the other special sensory systems, olfactory, gustatory and labyrinthine. Unimodal convergence also occurs in the cutaneous mechanoreceptive system of the dorsal columns and medial lemniscus. This can be seen by comparing the sizes of the peripheral cutaneous fields from which excitation can be evoked at various levels of the nervous system. For example, the average size of peripheral fields in the cat forelimb which can excite single dorsal root fibres is about 20 mm^2; while relay cells in the intermediate part of the dorsal column nucleus can be excited from a skin area of about 2000 mm^2. From this it can be deduced that about 100 primary afferent fibres, travelling in the dorsal columns, converge onto a single cell in the dorsal column nuclei.

Somatic Sensation

Nerve endings in the skin may be free, or may be encapsulated in some sort of specialized organule; they may be thick or they may be thin. These nerve endings are very numerous, and they form a plexus in the deeper layers of the skin, and are specific receptors for the types of sensation which can be appreciated by the skin. It should be emphasized here that all normal stimuli excite a large number of nerve endings, never just a single one.

The largest afferent fibres associated with sensory units in the skin and subjacent tissues come from pressure-sensitive Pacini corpuscles—which when synchronously activated in phase, as they can be in periosteum, give rise to vibration sensation. Other low threshold mechanosensory receptors, responsible for touch-pressure submodalities, also have large fibres (Group II or Aβ), as do the endings in joint capsules. Some articular sensory units are rapidly adapting, some are slowly adapting; some show spontaneous resting activity, while others discharge only during movement (see Chapter 5, page 40).

Smaller fibred (Group III or Aδ) sensory units comprise both high-threshold mechanoreceptors (including pricking receptors) and thermoreceptors, responsible for sensations of warmth and cold.

Unmyelinated (C or Group IV) primary afferents form free nerve endings in skin and most deep tissues, including viscera. In man, they seem practically all to belong to the category known as **polymodal nociceptors** which means they can be excited by high-energy mechanical and thermal (burning), as well as by chemical (e.g. stinging nettles) stimuli; they are responsible for slow, second, or real pain sensation. Many physiologists believe that since all the stimuli which activate polymodal nociceptors cause tissue damage, the true and unitary stimulus for these sensory units is a substance liberated from damaged cells.

Once these impulses reach the spinal cord, they are segregated according to modality. Impulses which will eventually be interpreted as the low-threshold mechanoreceptive sensations of touch, pressure, and kinaesthesia travel rostrally, without synapse in the cord, in the **dorsal columns** of the side on which they enter, after giving off a collateral to the grey matter of the dorsal horn in the segment of entry (Fig. 42). The long ascending branch of this first neurone of the low-threshold mechanosensory pathway ends in the **gracile** (leg and lower trunk) **cuneate** (arm and upper trunk) **nuclei** of the medulla oblongata. From here the second neurone travels to the thalamus. Efferent fibres from the dorsal column (gracile and cuneate) nuclei decussate by passing ventromedially in the medulla as **internal arcuate fibres,** and then pass rostrally as the **medial lemniscus.** In the medulla, the medial lemnisci lie between the olives (Fig. 22) but in the pons, rostral to the olive they lie in the ventral part of the tegmentum, just above the transverse pontine fibres and nuclei pontis (Fig. 24). In the midbrain (Figs. 26 and 27), the medial lemnisci occupy a more lateral position in the tegmentum, and as the fibres pass up into the diencephalon, they terminate in the lateral part of the **ventro-posterior nucleus** of the **thalamus.** Mechanoreceptor primary afferent fibres from the face and anterior part of the scalp terminate in the **principal sensory trigeminal nucleus,** which, although situated in the pons (Fig. 24), may be regarded as structurally and functionally homologous with the gracile and cuneate (dorsal column) nuclei. Efferent fibres from the principal sensory trigeminal nucleus, after decussation, join the (pontine) medial lemniscus and end in the medial part of the thalamic ventroposterior nucleus. Both parts of the ventroposterior nucleus project in an orderly fashion to the **post-central gyrus** (Fig. 40), such that the contralateral half of the body is represented upsidedown in each postcentral gyrus. The postcentral gyrus is known

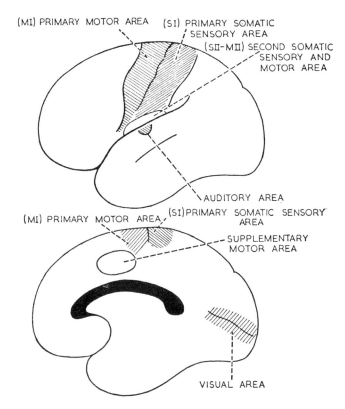

FIG. 40. Primary motor and sensory areas of the cortex. Above: lateral view. Below: medial view. Compare with the thalamo-cortical projection zones (Fig. 47).

as the **first somatic sensory area** (**SI**). Between the lower end of the central sulcus and the lateral fissure lies a **second somatic sensory area** (**SII**), on which sensations from the body are represented bilaterally, instead of unilaterally as in the main sensory area.

Two facts should be observed with regard to the mechano-receptive pathway. First, it is completely crossed (by the decussation of the medial lemnisci), so that all impulses travelling by this route end up in the postcentral gyrus of the side opposite to which the stimulus was originally applied. Second, strict somato-topical localization is maintained throughout the chain of three neurones. Thus, in the dorsal column of the cord, the lowermost fibres are most medially placed, the highest most laterally. In the (pontine) medial lemniscus, impulses generated in the feet are found travelling in the most laterally-placed fibres, those from the neck in the most medial axons. This arrangement is maintained in the ventroposterior thalamic nucleus, where the half body may be imagined lying horizontally with its foot against the internal capsule and its neck pointing medially. The arrangement in the postcentral gyrus is such that the half body is hanging upside-down, its knee bent over the supero-medial border of the hemisphere, and the foot going down on to the medial surface; however, the face, represented below the neck, is the right way up. Note that the amount of cortex allotted to representation of various body parts does not accord with their actual size, but with the relative richness of their sensory nerve supply. Thus the area occupied by the hand, for example, is very much greater than that occupied by the trunk. In the second somatosensory area, the distortion of the body surface is less marked than in the case of the first.

The primary afferent fibres which reach the gracile and cuneate nuclei in the dorsal columns belong to Group II or $A\beta$. Transmission through the dorsal column nuclei occurs, at least partially, by way of interneurones (Fig. 41). This kind of arrangement, whereby one cell is excited while its neighbours are inhibited through interneurones (b), leads to 'sharpening of the image', to increase topical localization of the point of maximal peripheral stimulation. It is known as **surround** or **collateral inhibition,** and may serve to restrict the peripheral receptive field of the thalamically-projecting cell (c) as much as eightfold compared with that of the primary relay neurone (a). Further discriminatory control, of the feedback variety, is exerted by fibres descending to the dorsal column nuclei from the sensorimotor cortex. These descending afferents excite the inhibitory interneurones (b) and inhibit the cells of origin of the medial lemniscus (c).

The fibres of the medial lemniscus, joined by functionally similar fibres originating in the principal sensory nucleus of the trigeminal nerve, terminate in the ventroposterior nucleus in an

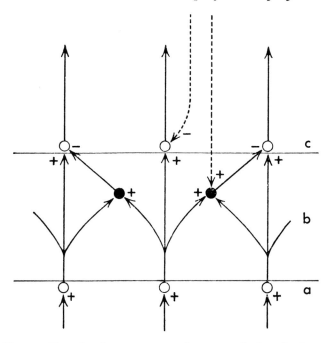

FIG. 41. Functional arrangement of neurones in dorsal column
nuclei. Caudal cells (row a) are excited by ascending fibres of
dorsal columns. Axons from these cells excite rostral cells in
row c; but axon collaterals excite inhibitory interneurones
(black) in middle row b. These in their turn inhibit neighbour-
ing cells in rostral row c (which transmit to the thalamus as
the medial lemniscus), thereby sharpening the image (lateral,
collateral, or surround inhibition). Descending fibres (interrupted lines) inhibit rostrally projecting cells in row c and
excite inhibitory interneurones in row b.

orderly somatotopic fashion. But this thalamic nucleus also receives ascending (**neospinothalamic**) fibres from cells in the
spinal grey matter (see Chapter 6), and analogous afferents
originating in the spinal (descending) trigeminal nucleus, which is
in direct continuity with the dorsal horn of the spinal grey matter.
Neospinothalamic fibres ascend in the anterolateral quadrant of
the spinal cord; after passing dorsolateral to the inferior olive in
the lower brainstem, they join the superolateral end of the medial
lemniscus in the pons and continue with it through the midbrain

into the thalamus. The spinal quintothalamic fibres also join the medial lemniscus. The neospinothalamic and spinal quinto-thalamic fibres (Fig. 42), although ending somatotopically in the thalamus differ in several ways from those of the medial lemniscus.

First, the primary peripheral afferent fibres (belonging mainly to Aδ or Group III) which reach their cells of origin come not only from tactile receptors (but NOT from hairs, Pacini corpuscles, or joints), but also from thermal and pinprick (*first* or *rapid pain*)* receptors. It is believed that the cells differentiate between these sensory submodalities by responding with a different spatio-temporal firing pattern according to the type of stimulus.

Secondly, these fibres are not all crossed in the spinal cord, some reaching the brain stem before gaining the side contralateral to their origin. Those neospinothalamic fibres which do decussate in the spinal cord take some 5 or 6 segments to do so.

Thirdly, this system, unlike that of the dorsal columns and medial lemniscus, does not exhibit surround inhibition. This, together with the fact that neospinothalamic fibres are some ten-fold fewer in number than those of the dorsal columns, accounts for the much larger size of neospinothalamic as compared with dorsal column peripheral receptive fields.

From the relay in the thalamic ventroposterior nucleus, which also receives feedback fibres from the somatomotor cortex, impulses are projected to the first (SI) and second (SII) cortical somatosensory areas. SI appears principally to reflect activity in the dorsal column-medial lemniscus (and associated principal trigeminal) system, in that it responds only to mechanical (includ-ing joint) stimulation of the contralateral half of the body and shows surround inhibition. SII, on the other hand, responds al-most exclusively to skin stimulation alone, from both sides of the body, and does not show much surround inhibition; thus it seems mainly to reflect activity in the neospinothalamic and associated spinal trigeminal systems.

* It should be noted that the unmyelinated (C or Group IV) sensory units formed by the polymodal nociceptors appear to be connected centrally with non-specific afferent systems (see Chapter 11).

Some proprioceptive information also reaches consciousness. This is believed to occur through collaterals of the dorsal and ventral spinocerebellar tract fibres which synapse in a relay nucleus in the medulla oblongata. Further fibres pass thence to the thalamus, and a final relay projects to the primary somatosensory cortex in the depths of the central sulcus.

The organization of the **specific auditory system** shows many similarities to, but some important differences from, that of the somatic pathway. Primary afferent neurones (each connected with only a single receptor) pass to the brainstem in the acoustic division of the eighth nerve. Like the vestibular division, the ganglion cells of these neurones are bipolar, rather than pseudo-unipolar, in accordance with their evolutionary antiquity. Acoustic axons bifurcate in order to establish connection with both **dorsal** and **ventral cochlear nuclei** (Fig. 23). The dorsal cochlear nucleus is extremely complex in structure; not only do entering primary afferents **diverge** on to its numerous cells, but it also contains many interneurones. Processes akin to surround inhibition occur at this level.

Secondary fibres arise from both cochlear nuclei, and many of them pass to the opposite side of the brain stem at the level of the ponto-medullary junction as the **trapezoid body**. The trapezoid body contains several scattered groups of nerve cells (the trapezoid nuclei) in which some, but by no means all, secondary auditory fibres undergo a further relay. Just rostral to the trapezoid body, in either side of the lateral part of the brainstem, lies a somewhat larger grey mass, the nucleus known as the **superior olive**, in which some fibres from the cochlear and trapezoid nuclei terminate. At this level the main body of the higher-order auditory fibres pass rostralward as the **lateral lemniscus**.

Two points should be noted at this juncture. The first is that while some secondary cochlear fibres decussate in the trapezoid body, others do not, with the result that each lateral lemniscus contains fibres conveying impulses generated in the organs of Corti of both sides. Secondly, there are neurones in the superior olivary nucleus which project to the peripheral receptor cells (olivo-cochlear bundle) thereby exerting feed-back control on the peripheral receptor organ itself. This is as yet the only known example in the mammalian nervous system, although the γ-efferent motoneurones supplying the receptor-containing intrafusal muscle fibres play a very similar role.

As the lateral lemniscus passes rostrally in the brain stem, it lies at first lateral to the medial lemniscus; but as it approaches the midbrain, it comes to lie dorsal to it. Most of its fibres terminate in the **inferior colliculus**, whence, by a further relay, they pass in the **brachium of the inferior colliculus** to the **medial geniculate body** (nucleus) of the thalamus (Fig. 29). Some fibres, however, pass through the inferior colliculus without interruption straight on to the medial geniculate body.

In addition to its projection to the medial geniculate body, some fibres from the inferior colliculus pass to the inferior colliculus of the other side, forming a further decussational linkage. Yet other efferents from the inferior colliculus run to cervical segments of the spinal cord, as a contingent of tecto-spinal fibres. This connection is responsible for reflex head turning in response to auditory stimuli.

Axons from the medial geniculate body are projected in a point-to-point fashion to the primary **auditory cortex** in the **superior temporal gyrus** (Fig. 40). This projection is tonotopic, such that different pitches of sound are represented in discrete regions of the auditory cortex. Experimental work on animals has indicated the presence of a second (and even third) auditory area in the cortex. It will be evident from what has been said above that every impulse generated in the organ of Corti will reach the auditory cortex by a number of routes, with a varying number of intercalated synapses; thus a single impulse in a primary afferent fibre will give rise to a burst of impulses, spread out in time, at higher levels of the auditory system. It should be noted that although impulses from one organ of Corti reach the primary auditory cortex of both sides, in functional terms the auditory projection is predominantly crossed.

Fibres from the **vestibular apparatus**, travelling in the **vestibular division of the eighth nerve**, terminate in all four of the **vestibular** group of **nuclei** (Fig. 25). Secondary connections exist between these nuclei and the cerebellum (see Chapter 14), and with the spinal cord as the vestibulospinal tract, arising from the lateral vestibular nucleus. Other fibres from the vestibular nuclei pass in the **medial longitudinal fasciculus** (Figs. 22, 23, 24, 26 and 27), by means of which they are distributed rostrally to the motor nuclei of the extrinsic eyeball muscles (III, IV, VI), and caudally to the hypoglossal nucleus (XII).

The pathways by which information from the vestibular apparatus reaches consciousness in the cerebral cortex are not well known. However, the cortical vestibular areas appear to be in the vicinity of the auditory area, while the thalamic relay is in the medialmost (magnocellular) part of the medial geniculate body, in the corner between the auditory relay and the somatic ventroposterior nucleus. Given that the Pacinian corpuscles, impulses from which relay in this latter nucleus, are low frequency vibration receptors, this means that in the caudalmost part of the ventral thalamic nuclear group, there is a latero-medial array of synapses transmitting high (sound), medium (vestibular), and low (Pacinian) frequency vibratory information.

Our knowledge of the secondary connections of **taste** fibres is also woefully incomplete. The primary afferent fibres, travelling in the VIIth (chorda tympani), IXth and Xth nerves, end in the rostral part of the **nucleus** of the **solitary tract.** Thence impulses are relayed, presumably by some part of the ventral thalamic nuclear complex, probably to a part of the **insular** cortex.

In the **visual system**, the first series of transformations, such as surround inhibition, are effected in the retina itself, which belongs therefore partly to the central nervous system. The layer of bipolar cells, onto which the photoreceptors project, corresponds to the primary afferent neurones of other systems. The ganglion cell layer, forming the second relay, corresponds functionally to the dorsal column or cochlear nuclei, and so its efferent pathway, the optic nerve and tract, is the equivalent of the medial or lateral lemnisci. Stress should be laid upon the primacy of the visual system in man, in whom it accounts for 40 per cent of the total sensory input to the nervous system, in terms of afferent fibre numbers.

At the **optic chiasma,** situated on the ventral surface of the brain at the anterior extremity of the hypothalamus, the optic nerve undergoes partial decussation, such that fibres from the nasal half of the retina (including half the macula) cross, while the fibres from the temporal half of the retina (and macula) remain on their side of origin. Thus the left **optic tract** (as the fibres are called after their partial decussation) conveys impulses generated by light coming from the right half of the visual field, while the right tract is concerned with information from the left half of the visual field.

The optic tracts wind around the midbrain, deep in the groove between the cortex and brain stem, until they reach the **lateral geniculate body** of the thalamus (Fig. 29), in the six layers of which most of the fibres terminate in an orderly fashion. Some fibres, however, continue in a caudomedial direction, passing through the **brachium of the superior colliculus,** to terminate in the **superior colliculus** of the mesencephalic tectum (Fig. 27). The superior colliculus and the **pre-tectal** area just rostral to it are the seat of the autonomic **light** and **accommodation** reflexes, by which the size of the pupillary opening is controlled. The superior colliculus also projects to the motor nuclei to the IIIrd, IVth and VIth cranial nerves, and, through its component of the tectospinal pathway, to the cervical segments of the spinal cord. It is thus responsible for reflex movements of the eyeballs and head in response to visual stimuli.

Efferent fibres from the lateral geniculate nucleus pass, as the **optic radiation,** along the lateral wall of the posterior horn of the lateral ventricle, to reach the visual cortex, which is on either side of the **calcarine sulcus,** on the medial aspect of the occipital lobe (Fig. 40). Analogously to the other primary thalamocortical projections, that from the lateral geniculate body to the visual cortex is retinotopic. Second and third visual areas have been described in experimental animals, in which visual information is progressively elaborated, in the sense that receptive fields, although becoming spatially larger, also become more sophisticated in terms of stimulus shape and direction of movement. It has been shown, in both visual and somatosensory areas, that all six layers of the cortex are arranged in vertical columns with respect to peripheral receptive fields.

The great neocortical commissure, the **corpus callosum,** is functionally associated with the visual system from an evolutionary point of view. The number of fibres in the corpus callosum is directly proportional to the number of non-decussated fibres in the optic tract; yet the corpus callosum joins mirror image points in the neocortex of both hemispheres, except for the primary sensory areas, which lack transcallosal interconnections.

Primary sensory cortices (somatic, auditory, and visual) are characterized by a great development of the granular layers (II and IV) and a corresponding diminution of the pyramidal layers (III and V). The specific (point-to-point) afferent fibres from the thalamus end in the fourth layer, where they form the **outer stripe** of **Baillarger.** However, from a functional point of view, there is evidence to suggest, so far as the primary sensory thalamo-cortical projections are concerned, that each thalamic point is associated with a vertical column or cylinder of cortical cells, extending through all six layers. Thus, in the primary visual cortex, for example, neurones in the fourth layer signal the presence or absence of a stimulus on the appropriate part of the retina, while in other layers, complex cells respond to particular shapes in the receptive field, and hypercomplex cells respond to particular directions of movement (of particular shapes) in the field.

Non-specific (diffuse thalamo-cortical and commissural) fibres form the **inner stripe** of **Baillarger,** between layers V and VI. In the visual cortex, the inner stripe is lacking, and the only (specific) one, equivalent to the outer stripe, is here known as the **line** of **Gennari.**

Each of the primary sensory cortices has adjacent to it an area of **association cortex** (Fig. 47), which is concerned with the inter-pretation of the information which is signalled directly to the specific cortex. The association cortex of the somatosensory area lies behind the postcentral gyrus, occupying most of the rest of the parietal lobe. The visual association cortex lies on the lateral surface of the occipital lobe, while the auditory association cortex surrounds the primary auditory area, save dorsally, where it is cut off by the lateral fissure. In the association cortices, the cell laminae are of more equal thickness than in the primary sensory cortical areas.

As can be seen in Fig. 47, the somatosensory, auditory, and visual association cortices meet around the posterior end of the lateral fissure. On the dominant side (see Chapter 13) this region of mixed associations is specialized for understanding of the spoken and written word, and is known as the **sensory speech area** of Wernicke.

While the somatosensory association area of each side is concerned with the recognition of objects (see Chapter 12) in contact with the body, and particularly with the hand (**stereognosis**), more complex associational functions are asymmetrical. Thus the parietal lobe on the side on which speech is represented is responsible for logical functions such as the ability to calculate. On the other side the parietal association cortex subserves the **gestalt** recognition of the subject's own body image and of his image ("internal map") of the outside world. Similarly, the auditory association area on the side not concerned with language is better at the non-analytical recognition of familiar tunes.

The visual association area occupies so much cortex that although a part of it is specialized on one side for recognition of the written word, there are no other discernible functional differences in visual recognition between the two sides.

CHAPTER ELEVEN

The Non-Specific Afferent System

Primitive vertebrates, although possessing some highly-developed special sense systems, do not have any organized somatic afferent systems such as those described in the preceding chapter; yet it is a commonplace observation that these animals react to somatic stimulation. The system which allows for integrated reactions of this type is a **non-specific afferent system**; non-specific because it can be shown to be activated by many different kinds of peripheral stimulation—indeed by all kinds of external energy for which appropriate receptors exist. It may therefore be deduced that a hypothetical ancestral vertebrate which did not possess *any* special sense systems would still have been the proud owner of a non-specific afferent system to which all its receptors would have been hooked up.

This primitive system persists in all higher vertebrates, including ourselves, and indeed is more essential to survival than the specific systems just discussed. The specific systems, being of more recent evolutionary origin, tend to overlay and conceal the older non-specific systems. The newer specific systems are sometimes, for brevity, called **lemniscal** systems; and so the non-specific system is called the **extralemniscal** system (compare **extrapyramidal system**, Chapter 13). It is also known as the **ascending reticular** or **reticular arousal system**. In concordance with the principle laid down in Chapter 4 the non-specific system is made up of neurones whose axons have a large number of collateral branches; these interweaving axons and collaterals, containing scattered (reticular) cells in their interstices, make up the primitive **neuropile**. Conversely, the newer systems are made up of neurones whose axons have few collateral branches.

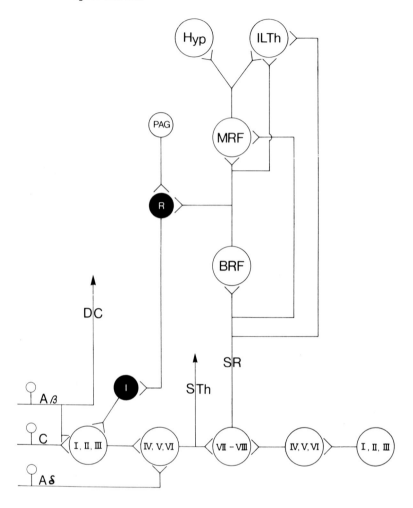

Fig. 42. Simplified schematic diagram of ascending reticular system. Inhibitory neurones are shown in black. Primary afferents are shown on the left, projecting to or through spinal grey laminae (Roman numerals—cf. Fig. 18). BRF: bulbar reticular formation; DC: dorsal columns; Hyp: hypothalamus; I: inhibitory enkephalinergic interneurone in substantia gelatinosa—it is not certain whether it can be activated directly by collaterals of Aβ primary afferents or whether the inhibition of C primary afferent input by Aβ primary afferent input (gate control) is indirect; ILTh: intralaminar thalamic

As can be seen in Fig. 42, the cells of origin of long (spino-reticular) extralemniscal fibres lie in the deep grey matter (laminae VII and VIII) of the spinal cord. They receive impulses which converge upon them from more superficial laminae, which in their turn are activated by primary peripheral afferents of Groups III and IV (Aδ and C); the effective peripheral stimuli are therefore of high intensity (though not necessarily painful) mechanical, including pinprick thermal, and polymodal nociceptive categories. Many neurones of laminae VII and VIII have bilateral receptive fields.

Fig. 42 also shows a segmental collateral of Group II (dorsal column) primary afferents entering lamina IV of the dorsal horn. These fibres are believed to be responsible for the presynaptic inhibition of impulses coming into the substantia gelatinosa. They thus form the morphological basis of the **gate control** mechanism whereby impulses in large fibres generated e.g. by gently rubbing the skin, partially block the transmission of information from polymodal nociceptors.

The longer spinal non-specific axons form the majority of ascending fibres in the antero-lateral white columns of the spinal cord, where they are mixed with a minority of neospinothalamic fibres. The non-specific extralemniscal fibres terminate either (a) at higher levels of the cord itself (spino-spinal or spinal reticular neurones), or (b) higher still on cells in the reticular formation of the brain stem (spino-reticular neurones), and finally, (c) a very small number carry right on up to the intralaminar nuclei of the thalamus (**palaespinothalamic fibres**). As ascending axons from the lower brainstem reticular formation also terminate in the intralaminar thalamic nuclei, these may be regarded as the rostral pole of the ascending reticular system (Fig. 43). A powerful contingent of axons ascending from the brainstem reticular formation also terminate in the hypothalamus and subthalamic regions.

nuclei; MRF: midbrain (mesencephalic) reticular formation; PAG: periaqueductal grey matter; R: serotoninergic descending inhibitory reticulospinal interneurone in brainstem raphe nuclei, whose axon descends in dorsolateral funiculus of spinal cord to activate inhibitory enkephalinergic interneurone I; SR: spinoreticular fibre; STh: spinothalamic fibre.

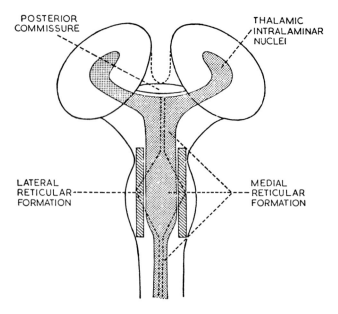

POSTERIOR
COMMISSURE

THALAMIC
INTRALAMINAR
NUCLEI

LATERAL
RETICULAR
FORMATION

MEDIAL
RETICULAR
FORMATION

FIG. 43. Diagram of the reticular formation projected on to a dorsal view of the brain stem and upper spinal cord. (Reproduced, by permission, from Bowsher, *Brit. J. Anaesth.*, 1961.)

The regions of the brainstem reticular formation in which spinoreticular fibres principally terminate are so arranged that they lie just caudal to reticular zones which send their axons downwards (reticulo-spinal neurones) (Fig. 44). In addition to the motor reticulo-spinal neurones (see Chapter 13), there are descending inhibitory controls (Fig. 42) arising from reticular cells in the midline raphe of the lower brain stem. By post-synaptic inhibition exerted in the spinal grey matter (Fig. 42), these raphespinal neurones are able to suppress, partially or completely, the upward transmission of information coming through the ascending non-specific system from the activation of small myelinated and un-myelinated primary peripheral afferents. Descending inhibitory raphespinal neurones are themselves activated by axons descending from a specialized region of the rostral brainstem reticular formation, the **periaqueductal** and **periventricular** grey matter (PAG in Fig. 42).

Tectoreticular (tectobulbar) fibres, originating in the superior and inferior colliculi, make synaptic contact with medullary reticular neurones, and therefore at this level convergence occurs between signals initiated by somatic stimuli and those initiated by visual and auditory stimuli. Many reticular neurones in this region have bifurcating axons, one branch of which passes up to the thalamic intralaminar nuclei while the other passes downwards to the spinal cord so that activity engendered by visual and auditory stimuli has an effect not only in the thalamus but also in the spinal cord.

The non-specific afferent, or ascending reticular, system will have been seen to be morphologically very complicated. Some of

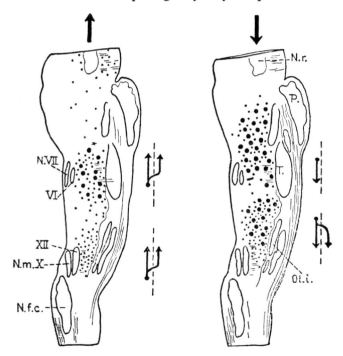

Fig. 44. Diagram of the grouping of ascending and descending reticular neurones in the brainstem of the cat, in lateral projection. (Reproduced, by permission, from Brodal, *The Reticular Formation of the Brain Stem*, Oliver & Boyd, Edinburgh, 1957.)

its features are diagrammatized in Fig. 45. However, it is important that certain features about the non-specific afferent system be clearly grasped:

1. Primary peripheral afferent fibres are common to both specific and non-specific systems, as are the first central neurones with which they synapse. Beyond the level of the first central neurone

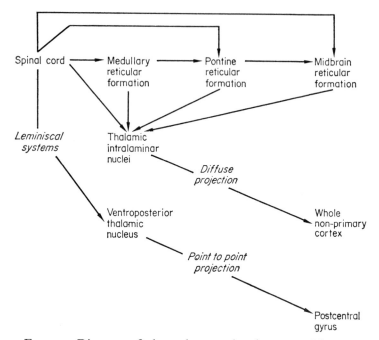

FIG. 45. Diagram of the point-to-point (somatotopic) so-matosensory pathway through the thalamus to the cortex, and the diffuse (reticular) pathway through the intralaminar nuclei. (Reproduced, by permission, from Bowsher, *Brit. J. Anaesth.*, 1961.)

bearing a long (specific) axon, however, both systems are com-pletely independent of one another; the ascending reticular system is **not** fired by collaterals from the specific (lemniscal) system at brainstem level.

2. The non-specific system should be thought of as the primitive central core of the neuraxial tegmentum, with very little sign of

lateralization. It is more helpful to think of it this way than to say, for example, that non-specific neurones on one side of the spinal cord project to cells on both sides of the medullary reticular formation, one side of which, in its turn, projects to the intralaminar nuclei of both thalami as well as bilaterally to the hypothalamus.

3. Although the central neurones of the non-specific system at the level of entry of primary afferents have short axons, at higher (organizational) levels, reticular neurones may have quite long axons with relatively restricted collateral branching. This is another way of saying that reticular neurones do not necessarily synapse with every other neurone in the vicinity of their trajectory, and that the non-specific system is really only non-specific in terms of place and modality. Even these properties may in some rather fuzzy way be encoded in the impulse patterns of the system.

4. Probably because of the interconnections between its excitatory and inhibitory neurones (Fig. 42), the ascending reticular system will only follow rates of peripheral stimulation up to 3 or 4 per second, compared with upwards of 100/sec for the specific systems.

The functions of the non-specific system may seem difficult to comprehend. Yet the fact that animals not possessed of specific somatic systems are to some extent capable of discriminating both site and modality of stimulation, presumably by a mechanism such as that mentioned in (3) above may yield a clue. The vital importance of the system in higher vertebrates can be demonstrated by animal experiment as well as by midbrain injuries in man. A critical experiment consists of destruction of the reticular core in the midbrain, while leaving the more laterally-placed specific auditory pathways (lateral lemnisci) intact. A loud noise can be registered as evoked potentials in the specific auditory cortex in such a preparation, while the animal remains resting and reacts in no way whatsoever to the stimulus. The contrary experiment, in which the lateral lemnisci are cut while the central reticular core is left intact, is even more instructive. In this case, the animal reacts violently to a loud noise, though electrodes on the specific auditory cortex show that the animal does not consciously 'hear' the sound at all. This of course is why the system is called an arousal system and it is evident from this kind of experiment that the integrity of both specific and non-specific systems, is necessary for both the conscious appreciation and identification of a stimulus and the appropriate reaction to it; and that, from a very basic biological point of view, the latter is more important than the former.

The ascending reticular system is probably responsible for the translation of those sensory qualities known at one time as 'protopathic'—poorly defined, poorly localized, and graduable, running the whole gamut from itch to agony. Because of their interconnections and lack of synaptic security, the quality of protopathic sensation realized in the cerebrum is most likely to be a function of the number of reticular neurones activated, the highest proportion representing (*second, slow* or *true*) pain. Indeed, the transmission of impulses bilaterally to the whole cerebral cortex which will be interpreted as true pain is, medically speaking, perhaps the most significant function of the ascending reticular system. The latter should be contrasted with the specific lemniscal systems where both place and modality (or submodality) depend on the activation not of a variable number, but of a particular set, of neurones.

The intralaminar thalamic nuclei project in a point-to-point fashion to the corpora striata (see Chapter 12); but they also project to the whole non-primary cortex. This is what is known as the 'diffuse thalamo-cortical projection', and is responsible for cortical arousal, not only in the sense implied in the preceding paragraph, but also electrically. Indeed, the electrical 'activation' of the cerebral cortex resulting from stimulation of the intralaminar thalamic nuclei is one of the best understood phenomena of electroencephalography (EEG).

In the normal awake but inattentive adult, synchronous summated rhythmic activity can be recorded across the cranium and scalp from the non-primary cortex at the rate of 8–12/sec; this is known as the α-rhythm. From the primary (pre- and post-central) cortex under the same conditions is recorded the β-rhythm of 18–32/sec. Any form of cerebral activity, varying from performing mental arithmetic with the eyes shut to admiring the electroencephalographist with the eyes open, causes general cortical arousal such that the resting rhythms are replaced by asynchronous, fast, low-voltage (because not summated) activity. None of these rhythms, synchronous or asynchronous, are an inherent property of the cortex, for they disappear in cortex isolated from the thalamus; they are transmitted to the cortex from the intralaminar nuclei of the thalamus. It is now known that the electroencephalogram can be changed, both towards as well as away from synchrony, by stimulation, at different rates, not only of the intralaminar thalamic nuclei, but also of lower levels of the ascending reticular system. It will be recalled (Chapter 7) that some parts of the lower brainstem reticular formation are spontaneously active; and this is also true of the higher, thalamic, levels of the system. A simple mechanical model of the non-specific core of the neuraxis would not be represented by a static wheel which is rotated in one direction or the other by the force of external events. Rather it should be seen as a wheel rotating at a regular intrinsic rate, which can be speeded up or slowed down (i.e. desynchronized) as a result of external changes.

CHAPTER TWELVE

Thalamic Projection to Telencephalon: Association

The consideration of sensory pathways in the preceding chapter has shown that they all relay through thalamic nuclei to the cortex. Thus somatosensory fibres (medial lemniscus, spinothalamic tract, and trigemino-thalamic tract) pass to the ventroposterior nucleus; the lateral (auditory) lemniscus to the medial geniculate body; and the optic tract to the lateral geniculate body. These three nuclei all belong to the **ventral nuclear complex** of the thalamus. To complete this, we may add the **ventrolateral** (and **ventro-anterior**) **nuclei,** which receive fibres from the cerebellum, red nucleus and globus pallidus.

The nuclei of the ventral complex have two important points in common, which are shared by no other thalamic nuclei. They all receive their afferent fibres from outside the thalamus, and they project somatotopically, tonotopically, or retinotopically to the primary motor and sensory areas of the cortex. The ventral complex is one of the six chief nuclear groups of the thalamus (Fig. 46). Lateral to the thalamus lies the internal capsule; it is separated from the thalamus by the **external medullary lamina**. Adjacent to this lamina, as a thin shield of cells bounding the whole lateral aspect of the thalamus, lies the **thalamic reticular nucleus,** which belongs developmentally to the ventral thalamus (subthalamus and zona incerta).

The interior of the thalamus is divided by the diagonally-placed **internal medullary lamina**. Rostrally, this splits to enclose the **anterior thalamic nuclei**; externally, they form the **anterior tubercle** of the thalamus. They receive afferents from the fornix (rhinencephalon) and mammillary bodies of the posterior hypothalamus via the mammilo-thalamic tract, and they project to the **cingulate gyrus** in a point-to-point fashion. Behind the anterior

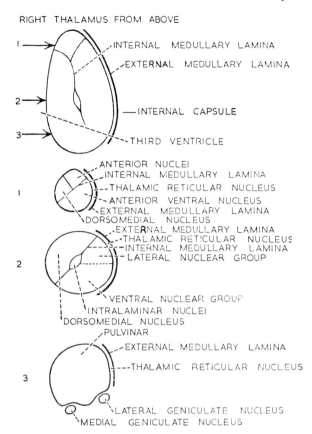

RIGHT THALAMUS FROM ABOVE

INTERNAL MEDULLARY LAMINA

EXTERNAL MEDULLARY LAMINA

INTERNAL CAPSULE

THIRD VENTRICLE

ANTERIOR NUCLEI
INTERNAL MEDULLARY LAMINA
THALAMIC RETICULAR NUCLEUS
ANTERIOR VENTRAL NUCLEUS
EXTERNAL MEDULLARY LAMINA
DORSOMEDIAL NUCLEUS
EXTERNAL MEDULLARY LAMINA
THALAMIC RETICULAR NUCLEUS
INTERNAL MEDULLARY LAMINA
LATERAL NUCLEAR GROUP

VENTRAL NUCLEAR GROUP
INTRALAMINAR NUCLEI
DORSOMEDIAL NUCLEUS
PULVINAR
EXTERNAL MEDULLARY LAMINA

THALAMIC RETICULAR NUCLEUS

LATERAL GENICULATE NUCLEUS
MEDIAL GENICULATE NUCLEUS

FIG. 46. Top: Diagram of the thalamus seen from above. 1, 2 and 3 are coronal sections through the thalamus at the levels indicated in the upper diagram.

nuclei, the large **dorsomedial** nucleus lies medial to the internal medullary lamina. This receives fibres from outside the thalamus and projects point-to-point to the cortex of the frontal lobe.

Two groups of nuclei lie lateral to the internal medullary lamina. Laterally and below is the ventral group, which has already been described. Above the ventral group is the **lateral group**. Caudal to the ventral nuclei, the internal medullary lamina moves medially and fades away. Thus the whole of the posterior part of the thalamus above the geniculate bodies is occupied by the largest of the lateral group of nuclei, the pulvinar. It is therefore convenient to refer to this whole group as the lateral-pulvinar complex. These nuclei are distinguished by receiving their afferents mainly from the specific (ventral) group of nuclei within the thalamus, although at least one of them, the lateral posterior nucleus, receives extrathalamic afferents as well, from the superior colliculus. They project in a point-to-point fashion to the **association areas** of cortex in the parietal and occipital lobes.

Lastly, there is a group of nuclei lying within the internal medullary lamina, and therefore known as the **intra-laminar nuclei**. Their connections are rather complicated, but both afferent and efferents can be divided into two groups. Afferents come from (a) outside the thalamus, from the ascending reticular system and fornix, and (b) within the thalamus, from other nuclei. Their efferent projections are (a) point-to-point, to the corpus striatum (caudate nucleus and putamen) and (b) diffuse to the whole nonprimary cortex (Chapter 11). At the caudal end of the thalamus, the intralaminar nuclei become continuous with certain ill-defined cell groups just medial to the medial geniculate body. Through this they become structurally, as well as functionally, continuous with the ascending reticular neurones of the midbrain tegmentum (Fig. 43).

A summary of the five point-to-point projecting groups shows that, with the exception of certain areas in the temporal lobe, the whole neocortex and the corpus striatum receive specific fibres from the thalamus (see table opposite).

Thus the whole telencephalon, except some of the neocortex of the temporal lobe, can be regarded as an umbrella cover, whose hub is the thalamus and the spokes of which are the specific point-to-point thalamo-telencephalic projections (Fig. 47). It can be seen from this that the true definition of a functional cortical area depends not upon the fortuitous folding of its surface into sulci and gyri, nor upon its cytoarchitecture (though this is related), but upon its specific projection from a particular thalamic nucleus. For example, the primary somatosensory cortex (roughly defined as the postcentral gyrus) is, in precise terms, only and entirely that area of cortex which receives its specific projections from the ventroposterior nucleus of the thalamus. Primary motor and sensory areas, as well as the hypothalamic-rhinencephalic areas of neocortex, are easily understood as those cortical areas which receive their specific projections from thalamic nuclei whose afferents are extra-thalamic. The parieto-occipital association areas, on the other hand, receive their specific projections from thalamic nuclei whose afferents are intrathalamic and tectal (lateral-pulvinar group). Specific thalamo-cortical fibres may be

	Afferents	Thalamic nuclei	Efferents
Extra-thalamic	Rhinencephalon and mammillary bodies	Anterior group	Cingulate gyrus
	Cell Groups in efferent and afferent hypothalamic pathways	Dorsomedial nucleus	Orbito-frontal (frontal lobe) cortex
	Cerebellum, globus pallidus Specific sensory pathways	Ventral group	Primary motor and sensory cortex
	Ascending reticular system Other thalamic nuclei	Intralaminar group	Corpus striatum Whole non-primary cortex
Intra-thalamic	Other thalamic nuclei Superior colliculus	Lateral-pulvinar group	Association cortex of parietal and occipital lobes

seen to terminate in the fourth layer of the cortex, where they are known as the outer stripe of Baillarger.

The non-auditory neocortex of the temporal lobe is also an association area, but unlike those in the parietal and occipital lobes, it is not thalamically dependent, though it does in fact receive a sparse projection from the pulvinar. However, it is connected to the parietal and occipital association areas by (relatively) long cortico-cortical fibres, known as **association bundles**. Just as there are two kinds of association cortex—thalamically-dependent (parietal and occipital) and independent (temporal), so is the mental act of association a double process. Anatomically, it can be represented:

Cortex	Primary sensory area	Parieto-occipital association area →	Temporal association area

Cortex — Primary sensory area — Parieto-occipital association area → Temporal association area

↑ (below Primary sensory area) ↑ (below Parieto-occipital)

Thalamus — Ventral nucleus → Lateral nucleus

↑ (below Ventral nucleus)

Brain Stem — Extrathalamic sensory pathway

The first associative act, occurring in the parieto-occipital or superior temporal thalamically-dependent association cortices, is essentially **cognitive**—that is, it tells us what it is we feel or see or hear. In the non-thalamically-dependent temporal neocortex, these cognitions are associated with other experiences, which may be simultaneous, or may be remembered from the past, and **interpreted**. Memory 'patterns' seem to exist principally in the temporal lobe, though not only in the cortex; they are dependent to some extent upon the connections of the non-auditory temporal neocortex with rhinencephalic structures (Chapter 15).

The thalamic intralaminar nuclei project in a diffuse (i.e. not point-to-point) manner to the whole non-primary cortex. These fibres end between the fifth and sixth layers, as the inner stripe of Baillarger. The intralaminar nuclei represent the rostral end of the ascending reticular system and receive fibres from the lower parts thereof. As most peripheral stimuli cause impulses to be fired into this system, the anatomical arrangement of the diffuse projection ensures that the whole cortex is 'aroused' in a non-specific manner by any stimulus whatsoever. If this were not so, there would be no response to specific stimuli arriving in the primary sensory and association areas.

The arousal effect is in addition to, though concomitant with, the vehiculation by the diffuse thalamocortical projection of impulses consciously interpreted as 'protopathic' sensory experiences, particularly second or true pain (see Chapter 11).

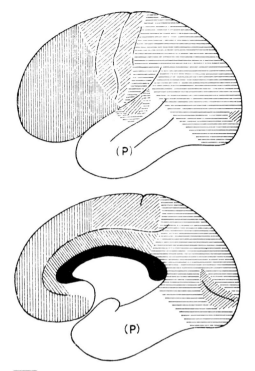

▨ Ventral group (primary motor and sensory cortex)

▨ Anterior nuclei (projection from mammillary bodies and hippocampus)

▥ Dorsomedial nucleus (hypothalamic projection zone)

▤ Lateral-Pulvinar group (cognitive association cortex)

[(P)] Non-thalamically dependent cortex, with some projections from pulvinar
(interpretive association cortex)

FIG. 47. Projection zones of the specific thalamic nuclei on the cerebral cortex. Above: lateral view. Below: medial view. Compare with Fig. 40.

CHAPTER THIRTEEN

Skeletal Motor Systems

In the light of what has been said in the last chapter, the **motor cortex** is properly defined as the cortical projection area of the ventrolateral nucleus of the thalamus (Fig. 47). Within this area, three different functional regions can be recognized (Fig. 40). Chief of these is the **main** or **principal motor area** which occupies the pre-central gyrus. Here also the body is represented upside-down, as in the sensory area, but with certain differences in detail. Thus although the lower limb lies above the upper limb which lies above the face, the axial (trunk) musculature is represented slightly anterior but parallel to the extremities. The motor cortex of the pre-central gyrus is sometimes known as **agranular cortex,** because the development of laminae III and V (especially the latter) is so great that the granular layers (II and IV) are almost non-existent in this type of cortex.

The principal motor area, like the corresponding sensory area, is carried over the supero-medial border of the hemisphere on to the medial surface, where the lower leg and foot find their representation. Just below and in front of the principal leg and foot area, on the medial surface, is the **supplementary motor area**; here the body is represented lying horizontally, head forwards. At the lower end of the central sulcus is the **second motor area.** It should be noted that this is co-extensive with the second sensory area (Chapter 10), so that it should really be known as the second motor **and** sensory area.

When a stimulus is applied to the principal motor area, a movement occurs in the appropriate part of the body on the contralateral side. Note that this is always a movement, i.e. the contraction of a certain muscle or group of muscles, accompanied by relaxation of its antagonists, and perhaps the concomitant contraction of its synergists—never just the uncoordinated contraction of a single muscle or group of muscles. Yet it is remarkable that in man, stimulation of the principal motor cortex has never been known to elicit movements of which a newborn baby is not capable; the mystery must lie deeper. Stimulation of the second motor area produces the same kind of results as does stimulation of the precentral gyrus, but it is necessary to use a stronger current in order to elicit the effects. Stimulation of the supplementary motor area brings about rather more complicated bilateral movements than stimulation of the precentral gyrus, but they are still simple, e.g. co-ordinated walking movements.

It will be the task of this chapter to follow fibres, or rather chains of fibres, from these cortical areas to the cells of the lower motor neurone, i.e. the motor cranial nerve or spinal anterior horn cells. Motor systems fall into two great categories: those which are somatotopically organized and subserve skilled movements (cortico-spinal and rubro-spinal); and those generally more diffusely organized systems concerned with the control of tone and posture, classically but wrongly known as extrapyramidal. We shall deal first with the simpler and (phylogenetically) more recently developed pyramidal system.

The fibres of this pathway arise from the fifth layer of the cortex, predominantly in the precentral gyrus (primary motor area); however some corticospinal axons are contributed by the parietal lobe (postcentral gyrus). After leaving the cortex, the fibres pass through the corona radiata and converge on the internal capsule (Fig. 36). In the genu of the internal capsule they show a definite orderly arrangement, with the lower limb area most posterior and the neck and face more anterior. These fibres then pass down into the cerebral peduncle, in the manner described in Chapter 6. Here they occupy the middle three-fifths of the basis pedunculi (Figs. 26 and 27), the lower limb fibres being most lateral and the face most medial, as would be expected from the manner in which the fibres of the internal capsule rotate into the basis pedunculi.

In the pons, the descending corticospinal tract is broken up into a number of small bundles by the transverse pontine fibres crossing at right angles to them. In this region (Fig. 24) of the brain stem those fibres of the pyramidal tract originating in the face area of the cortex terminate among the internuncial neurones surrounding the motor nuclei of the contralateral Vth and VIIth nerves, and also the nuclei of the extrinsic eyeball and tongue muscles (III, IV, VI, XII), and the nucleus ambiguus, which provides motor fibres to the trapezius and sternomastoid muscles, and the muscles of the palate, pharynx and larynx which are derived from branchial arch mesoderm.

In the medulla oblongata (Fig. 22), the remaining pyramidal fibres occupy the ventral zone of the brain stem, causing an external prominence known as the medullary pyramid. It is for this reason that the pathway is known as the pyramidal tract, **not** because it arises from pyramidal cells in the cortex. At the junction of the medulla and spinal cord, some 85 per cent of the pyramidal fibres turn dorsolaterally and cross the midline to occupy a position in the lateral white column of the opposite side of the cord (Fig. 21). This **pyramidal decussation**, as mentioned in Chapter 7, obliterates the anterior median sulcus at the spino-medullary junction. Thus in the cord there is a large crossed **lateral corticospinal** (pyramidal) **tract**, and a much smaller **anterior direct** (i.e. uncrossed) **corticospinal tract** (Fig. 16). The former runs the whole length of the cord, while the latter ends in the lower cervical or upper thoracic region. The fibres of the corticospinal tracts end mainly on interneurones in laminae IV, V, and VI of the spinal grey matter (Fig. 18), from which impulses are relayed to the motor cells of the anterior horn, whence the final **lower motor neurone** leads to striated musculature as the effector organ. Note that in segments whose motoneurones control movements of the digits, corticospinal fibres make direct (monosynaptic) contacts with the motoneurones (Lamina IX). Thus the corticobulbar and corticospinal pathways are made up of a chain of two or three neurones (Fig. 48). The first is long, leading from the cortex to the motoneurones or internuncial cells in the region of the motor cranial nerve nuclei or anterior horn cells; the second, not always present, is very short, being a neurone whose cell body is in the vicinity of the cranial motor nerve nucleus or anterior horn cell, and whose axon impinges upon one or other of these;

while the third is the lower motor neurone, consisting of the cells of the cranial motor nerve nuclei or spinal anterior horns, whose axons leave the neuraxis to reach, as motor peripheral nerves, the striated muscles upon which the pyramidal system has its effect.

The pyramidal motor system exerts its effects on willed or skilled or *fractionated* movements, while most reflex and postural movements are not under the influence of this system. Extirpation of the precentral gyrus alone causes a **flaccid paresis** of the **voluntary musculature**. Extirpation of the (non-pyramidal) supplementary motor area alone causes **spasticity** (hypertonia) of voluntary musculature, without paresis (apart from the awkwardness of movement caused by the spasticity). In human pathology it is more frequent to come upon lesions of the internal capsule, in which fibres from both sources (as well as many other non-pyramidal axons) are damaged. The result is a mixture of the symptoms described above, namely **spastic paresis**—always, of course, affecting the side of the body opposite the lesion. Section of the pyramidal tract in the cerebral peduncle, medulla or cord has surprisingly little effect, beyond producing a certain gaucheness of highly skilled movements.

There are a certain number of *pyramidal reflexes*, the normal functioning of which depends upon the integrity of the corticospinal tracts. These are the **abdominal reflex**—contraction of the muscles of the anterior abdominal wall on stroking the skin over it, the **cremasteric reflex** whereby the muscle of that name contracts on stroking the skin on the inner aspect of the thigh; and the **plantar reflex**, in which the big toe bends downwards on scratching the sole of the foot. In pyramidal lesions, the abdominal reflex is abolished, while the normal plantar reflex is replaced by the **Babinski (extensor plantar) reflex**, in which the big toe bends upwards on plantar stimulation, and all the toes splay out.

The pyramidal system is unique in that, in primates, some of its fibres make direct contact with the motoneurones which are responsible for fractionated movements of the digits. It is known that many of the interneurones with which pyramidal fibres make

synaptic contact are inhibitory to motoneurones, and are responsible for the reciprocal inhibition which is the invariable concomitant of pyramidal activity (Fig. 19). All other motor systems
descending to the spinal cord from higher levels end in contact
with interneurones, which may be either excitatory or inhibitory
in their action on motoneurones, or with motoneurone dendrites
extending beyond the confines of lamina IX. It must not be
imagined that non-pyramidal upper motor neurones (as the long
descending neurones are called) of different origin share the same
interneurones; each system has its specific group of interneurones.
These are so arranged, morphologically, that the more ancient,
phylogenetically, the upper motor neurone, the nearer the interneurones are placed to the motoneurones; i.e. the interneurones
mediating impulses from the most primitive descending motor
systems are situated ventrally, in the ventral grey horn, while
those of the most recently developed motor systems are situated
successively more dorsally in the dorsal horn (see Chapter 6).

In front of the precentral gyrus (area 4) lies a **motor co-
ordination area** (areas 6 and 8), sometimes known as the motor
association area, in which the body representation corresponds
more or less to that in the principal motor area behind it. Thus
for example opposite the upper face region of the precentral
gyrus is the **frontal eye field,** stimulation of which causes con-
jugate deviation of *both* eyes to the opposite side. While the frontal
eye fields are the same on both sides, other parts of the motor
co-ordination area are asymmetrical. Thus handedness is due to
greater development of the appropriate part of this cortical area on
the side opposite the dominant hand. Opposite the lower face
region of the principal motor area on one side (the left in 97% of
cases) is the **motor speech area** of Broca, which co-ordinates
movements of larynx, palate, tongue and lips, making speech
possible.

The role of the **rubro-spinal** system has been somewhat dis-
puted in the primate; however, the most recent evidence favours
its importance as a mediator of what might be called 'semi-
skilled' movements. Both the magnocellular and parvocellular
parts (and the latter predominates in primates) of the red nucleus

send their axons down into the spinal cord as the **rubrospinal tract** (Fig. 16); and it has been shown that the crossed rubrospinal projection is somatotopically organized. The principal cortical projection on to the parvocellular red nucleus comes from the supplementary motor area. These cortico-rubral fibres are bilaterally distributed, so that stimulation of the supplementary motor area brings about co-ordinated actions of both sides of the body, such as stepping movements.

The motor system classically known as **extrapyramidal** (Fig. 48) is that which is controlled by the **basal ganglia**. In fact, this system influences motor activity through its feedback control on other descending systems.

The neostriatum (caudate nucleus and putamen) receive their afferents from:

1. The whole cortex, in a radial fashion, so that, for example, the cortico-caudate projection would appear like the spokes of a three-dimensional wheel; physiological evidence indicates that this connection is largely inhibitory.

2. The intralaminar nuclei of the thalamus; this projection is organized in a point-to-point fashion, and appears to be mainly excitatory in function.

3. The substantia nigra (Fig. 30), whose cells contain melanin. The nigrostrial projection is dopaminergic.

The neostriatum sends fibres to the globus pallidus (palaeostriatum), which has a two-way connection with the subthalamus (Corpus Luysii). The cells of the neostriatum are both large and small, whereas those of the globus pallidus, substantia nigra, and subthalamus are uniformly large. The globus pallidus has two-way connections with the subthalamus (Fig. 48), but its principal discharge pathway is through the ansa and fasciculus lenticularis to the thalamus, where it sends fibres both to the nucleus centrum medianum of the intralaminar group, and to the lateral and anterior portions of the ventral group (which discharge to the motor cortex). ·

The centromedian thalamic nucleus projects not only to the neostriatum, but also diffusely to the whole cerebral cortex. Cortical axons project to the (descending) reticular formation.

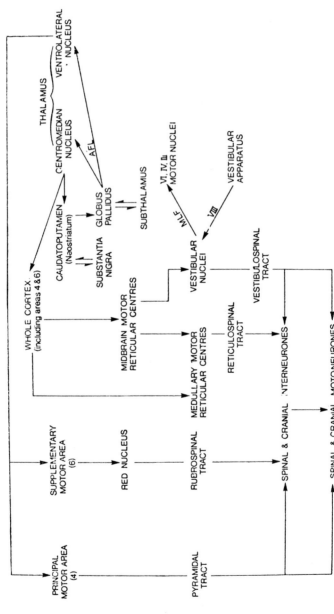

FIG. 48. Schematic diagram to show connections of motor systems controlling the activity of skeletal muscle. Note that the 'extrapyramidal system' (see text) works entirely through a feedback projection via the ansa and fasciculus lenticularis (AFL) to the thalamus and thence to the cortex, which then activates the motor reticular centres in the brainstem. The medial longitudinal fasciculus (MLF) also carries fibres (not shown) from the motor reticular

The mesencephalic part of the latter does not project beyond the lower brainstem, but neurones of the medial pontobulbar reticular formation give rise to **reticulospinal** pathways.

Within the brainstem reticular formation, neurones of the descending reticular system are arranged in blocks situated just rostral to those of the ascending reticular system (Fig. 44). Thus the axons of the descending and ascending systems pass through each other's dendritic fields, so that interaction is possible at each level. It should be noted that the cells of the lateral part of the reticular formation, situated in the medulla oblongata, project neither upwards nor downwards, but medially into the medial part of the reticular formation. Their action is to produce facilitation of motoneurones, by inhibiting those medial reticulo-spinal neurones which normally inhibit motoneurones. While, therefore, there is no direct lateral reticulo-spinal pathway, it is interesting to note that the **vestibulo-spinal** fibres, whose cells of origin have been, as it were, carved out of the lateral reticular formation, are also strongly facilitatory to motoneurones. The uncrossed vestibulospinal system, which under normal circumstances is tonically inhibited from specialized regions of the midbrain reticular formation (interstitial nucleus of Cajal), acts on antigravity muscles, which in man are chiefly the extensor muscles of the lower limbs. The lateral vestibular nucleus (of Deiters), which gives rise to vestibulospinal fibres, is excited by the saccule and utricle of the vestibular apparatus, which are sensitive to gravity.

Diseases of the so-called extrapyramidal system are characterized, as might be expected, by changes in muscular tone; and also by various kinds of 'spontaneous' movement, ranging from tremor to more or less violent writhing or jerking movements (athetosis, chorea, hemiballismus), presumably due to the release of the inhibition normally exerted by extrapyramidal structures.

The extrapyramidal system can be seen to be essentially a servomechanism, consisting of a number of interlinked feedback circuits. Its function is to regulate the output of other, more direct, motor systems. As will be seen in the next chapter, further feedback controls are exerted on central motor systems by the cerebellum.

The superior and medial vestibular nuclei, which are excited from the semicircular canals (sensitive to linear acceleration of the head), project through the medial longitudinal fasciculus (Chapter 7) to the nuclei of the third, fourth, and sixth nerves. This connection ensures co-ordination between head and eye movements.

CHAPTER FOURTEEN

The Cerebellum

In the preceding chapter, the cerebellum was introduced as part of a feedback circuit governing the activity of the extrapyramidal motor system. As in fact the whole function of the cerebellum is in mechanisms of this sort, it is convenient to consider it at this juncture. Its topographical anatomy must first be described.

The cerebellum lies above the medulla and pons, occupying the greater part of the posterior cranial fossa. It can be seen to be attached to the brain stem by three **peduncles** (Fig. 25), made up of nerve fibres, on each side. The largest and most superficial of these is the wide **middle peduncle**, or **brachium pontis** (Figs. 23 and 24), passing between the cerebellum and the pons; the trigeminal nerve emerges from the middle of this peduncle. Just medial to the brachium pontis is the **inferior peduncle** or **restiform body** (Fig. 25). This consists of fibres passing between the medulla and cerebellum, which at first run rostrally on the lateral aspect of the dorsal surface of the medulla, and then, medial to the brachium pontis, turn sharply dorsalwards into the cerebellum. The smallest, medialmost and rostralmost of the three peduncles is the superior peduncle or **brachium conjunctivum** (Figs. 24 and 26). This band of fibres passes from the cerebellum rostro-ventrally into the brain stem at the junction of the pons and midbrain.

The space between the cerebellum above and the rostral medulla and pons below is the **fourth ventricle**. This is closed superiorly by a membrane, the **superior medullary velum**, stretched between the two brachia conjunctiva. Inferiorly too, a rather thinner membrane, the **inferior medullary velum**, stretches from the inferior aspect of the cerebellum to the medulla at the level of the dorsal column nuclei. A median aperture in the inferior medullary velum, the **foramen** of **Magendie**, allows the fourth ventricle to communicate with the subarachnoid space. The fact that man's reputed best friend, the horse, does not possess such a foramen, has led some anatomists erroneously to deny its existence in man.

The fourth ventricle also communicates with the subarachnoid space at its lateral extremity, where there is a small interval between the caudal border of the brachium pontis and the infero-rostral border of the inferior peduncle (Fig. 25). This is known as the **foramen** of **Luschka**, and a small tuft of the choroid plexus of the fourth ventricle can be seen protruding through it into the subarachnoid space.

When viewed from the dorsal aspect, the cerebellum can be seen to possess a median elevation, the **vermis**, on either side of which lie the (lateral) **lobes**. Intervening between the raised vermis and the lateral lobe proper is a narrow depression, which represents the **paravermal** or **intermediate zone** (q.v.). The cortex is folded, as in the cerebrum, but in a more orderly fashion. All the sulci run across the vermis and lobes, at right angles to the long axis of the brain stem. The intervening ridges of cortex are called **folia**. From superficial external examination, all the fissures seem to be of equal depth. In lateral view, a small piece of cerebellar cortex can be seen just behind the tuft of choroid plexus protruding from the foramen of Luschka. This is the **flocculus**, and can be seen to be separated by a cleft from the lobar cortex just behind it. In the separated cerebellum this fissure can be seen to run right across the base; it is the **posterolateral fissure**. In front of it are, laterally, the flocculus, and in the vermis, the associated **nodule**. The two together (for they are connected by a small stalk) make up the **flocculonodular lobe.**

Study of a median sagittal section through the cerebellum reveals that the whole organ is in fact twisted round so that it looks like the third letter of the alphabet lying on its side ($\cap$). Moreover, the fissures can now be seen to be of unequal depth. Near the front is the particularly deep **primary fissure**. If we imagine now the cerebellum unrolled and laid out flat (Fig. 49)

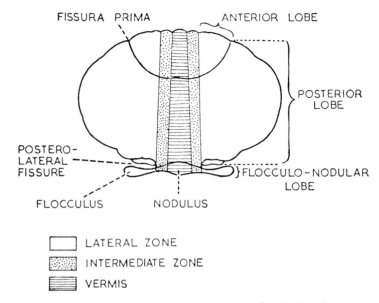

FIG. 49. Diagram of the cerebellum laid out flat, in dorsal view, to show the rostro-caudal and medio-lateral organization and divisions, and the cortico-nuclear projection.

then that part in front of the primary fissure is the **anterior lobe**; between the primary and postero-lateral fissures, the **posterior lobe**; and behind the postero-lateral fissure, the flocculonodular lobe. Fanciful names have been given to many other parts of the cortex and lateral lobes, but it is unnecessary for the student to learn these.

The cerebellar cortex is uniform throughout in its structure, and has only three layers. The middle layer consists of a single row of very large **Purkinje cells**. These have axons that lead away from the cortical surface, while their dendrites spread out in the opposite direction, to reach the superficial **molecular layer**. The Purkinje-cell dendritic tree is so arranged that it spreads out at right angles to the long axis of the folium (i.e. parallel with the vermis). Granular-type cells in the molecular layer have axons going in the same direction as Purkinje dendrites and which give off collateral branches that ensheath the Purkinje cells; because of this meshwork, they are called **basket cells**. The deepest layer is the **granular**, the axons of whose cells run peripherally into the molecular layer and then branch in a T-fashion, the branches running in the long axis of the folium (i.e. at right angles to the vermis). It will be seen that this arrangement provides for the greatest possible integration and interaction throughout the cerebellar cortex. Afferent fibres to the cortex end in the dendritic fields of the cells of the granular layer.

As in the case of the cerebral hemispheres, the cerebellum has nuclear masses deep in the white matter. The largest and most laterally placed of these nuclei is the **dentate nucleus**. Medial to this are the small **globose** and **emboliform nuclei** (often referred to collectively as the nucleus interpositus), and most medially is the **fastigial nucleus**. Most of the Purkinje cell axons terminate in these nuclei; and the projection is an exceedingly orderly one. Purkinje cells in the vermis project on the fastigial nucleus (Fig. 49), save for a few in the nodulus and anterior lobe vermis which go down through the inferior peduncle to the **vestibular nuclei**. On either side of the vermis is the paravermal (paramedian) zone, which projects on to the globose and emboliform nuclei; while the cortex of the lateral lobes, by far the largest zone, projects on to the dentate nuclei (Fig. 49).

All the afferent fibres to the cerebellum terminate in the cortex, some giving off collaterals to the cerebellar nuclei on the way. They come from three sources: the cerebral hemispheres and brain stem (descending afferents), the vestibular nuclei, and the spinal cord (ascending afferents). All the pathways of the first group and many of the third undergo synaptic interruption in the brain stem, so that secondary fibres are relayed to the cerebellum from centres receiving ascending and descending afferents.

Vestibular Afferents

A few primary vestibular fibres end not in the vestibular nuclei, but in the cortex of the flocculo-nodular lobe. There is a much larger projection of secondary fibres from the vestibular nuclei to the flocculonodular lobe cortex. A few of these fibres reach the anterior lobe vermis.

It may be noted that surgical removal of the nodulus abolishes the ability to experience motion sickness.

Descending Afferents

(a) Fibres arriving from the same area of the cerebral cortex as give rise to the pyramidal tract terminate in the **nuclei pontis** (Fig. 24), which are scattered throughout the basal part of the pons, in the interstices between the transverse pontine fibres and the descending pyramidal fibres. Secondary axons given off by these pontine cells travel first as **transverse pontine fibres,** and then pass up into the cerebellum as the **brachium pontis**. They are distributed to all parts of the cerebellar cortex except the flocculonodular lobe. While the hemispheres receive mainly crossed fibres, those to the vermis are both crossed and uncrossed.

It should be noted that while the vast majority of afferent fibres to the pontine nuclei descend from the cortex, a small number ascend from the spinal cord.

(b) The inferior olive (Fig. 22) receives descending fibres from higher levels of the 'extrapyramidal' motor system. The projection on to the olive is arranged in a point-to-point fashion. The largest number of olivary afferents come from the **red nucleus** and the grey matter surrounding the cerebral aqueduct in the midbrain— the **periaqueductal grey** (whose afferents probably come from the hypothalamus as well as the extrapyramidal system). These fibres from the mesencephalon descend to the olive as the **central tegmental tract**. Other descending afferents to the olive come from the 'extrapyramidal' areas of the cerebral cortex. As in the case of the pontine nuclei, the olive receives a few fibres ascending from the spinal cord.

Fibres arising in the olive stream across the medullary tegmentum as one group of **internal arcuate fibres** (the other group, it will be remembered, are the decussating efferents from the dorsal column nuclei), to enter the cerebellum via the inferior peduncle of the opposite side. Here they are distributed to the whole of the cerebellar cortex, including that of the flocculonodular lobe (although the olive receives no afferents from the vestibular nuclei). Those parts of the olive which project to the vermis of the anterior lobe receive their afferents from the spinal cord; the rest of the olive, receiving descending afferents, projects to the hemispheres and posterior lobe vermis.

Ascending Afferents

DIRECT

(a) The **dorsal spinocerebellar** tract arises at the root of the posterior horn in a group of large cells in the medial part of lamina VI between the second lumbar and lower cervical segments, known as the **column** of **Clarke** (Fig. 50). Primary afferent fibres to cells of the column of Clarke come from the muscle spindles (Group Ia), which are sensitive to lengthening or shortening of the muscle fibres in which they are situated; this information is known as **proprioception**. The secondary fibres arising in the column of Clarke form the dorsal spinocerebellar tract, and travel in the dorsolateral part of the spinal white matter, to ascend into the cerebellum through the inferior peduncle; they are distributed to the paravermal zone of the anterior and posterior lobe cortex. The dorsal spino-cerebellar fibres are the largest, and therefore the most rapidly conducting, in the human neuraxis. None of the fibres cross, either in their origin, course, or terminal distribution, so that the cerebellar cortex receives spino-cerebellar fibres from the same side of the body as that on which they enter.

(b) Those primary afferent fibres which terminate in the column of Clarke below the lower cervical region, above this level turn rostrally and terminate in the **external cuneate nucleus** (Fig. 25). This nucleus lies on the dorsal surface of the medulla, just lateral to the cuneate nucleus (with which it has no functional connection). Being in every way homologous with the column of Clarke, efferents from the external cuneate nucleus pass via the ipsilateral restiform body to the paravermal zone of the anterior and posterior lobe cortex.

(c) Fibres of the **ventral spino-cerebellar tract** arise from cells in the lateral part of lamina VI of the spinal grey matter. These axons cross immediately to the other side of the cord, where they ascend on the periphery of the lateral and anterolateral white column ventral to the dorsal spino-cerebellar fibres. However, they do not enter the inferior peduncle with these, but pass on up to the level of the midbrain, where they make a hairpin bend and turn back into the superior peduncle. After entering the cerebellum they are distributed bilaterally to the vermis and paravermal zones of the anterior and posterior lobes.

Primary proprioceptive afferents to separate cells of the column of Clarke and the external cuneate nucleus come from both muscle-spindle and Golgi tendon organs; those to the cells of origin of the ventral spino-cerebellar tract come exclusively from Golgi tendon organs (Group Ib). These are the only non-motoneurone terminations of these Group I primary afferent fibres; therefore all true proprioceptive information is principally relayed via the cerebellum (Fig. 50). Cells of origin of both spinocerebellar tracts are also activated directly or indirectly by cutaneous (but not articular) afferents, because of their convergent input from neurones of more superficial spinal laminae.

As has been mentioned in Chapter 10, collaterals of both dorsal and ventral spinocerebellar fibres relay in the medulla oblongata, whence their further projection to the thalamus and cortex is believed to be responsible for the conscious component of proprioception.

INDIRECT

In addition to their descending connections, which are the great majority, it has already been mentioned that both the olive and the pontine nuclei receive some ascending afferents from the spinal cord.

(a) In the ventrolateral medulla, just lateral to the olive, lies the **nucleus of the lateral funiculus** (Fig. 22) (sometimes called the lateral reticular nucleus). This nucleus receives fibres from the antero-lateral column of the cord by a point-to-point (somato-topical) projection. In its turn, this nucleus itself projects somato-topically to the cerebellar cortex, the fibres passing through the inferior peduncle. Some afferent fibres, particularly those to the medial part of the nucleus, do not come from the cord, but descend from higher levels of the brain stem. That part of the nucleus which receives fibres from the arm and leg segments of the

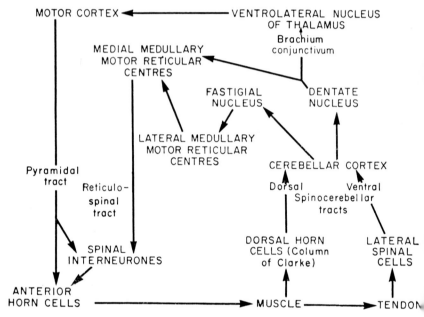

FIG. 50. Diagram to show the efferent connections of the cerebellum, together with its afferent proprioceptive input. The accessory brachium conjunctivum (from the fastigial nucleus) and the connections between the cerebellum and the lateral vestibular nucleus are not shown.

cord projects to the vermis, while that part receiving descending afferents projects to the lateral lobes (hemispheres). A third and rostrally placed part of the nucleus of the lateral funiculus, called the sub-trigeminal part, whose afferent connections are unknown, projects to the flocculonodular lobe.

(b) One or two other small nuclei in the medullo-cervical tegmentum, namely the **paramedian reticular nucleus**, between the emerging roots of the hypoglossal nerve, and other nearby, small, **peri-hypoglossal nuclei**, receive afferent fibres from the spinal cord and project through the inferior peduncle to the cerebellum.

It will have been noted that there is a tendency for impulses coming directly or indirectly from the trunk and limbs to project on to the vermis and paravermal (intermediate) zones of the anterior lobe, and to a lesser extent on the posterior lobe vermis; while impulses descending from higher levels of the nervous system are mainly projected on to the lateral lobes (hemispheres).

It has been seen that most ascending impulses to the cerebellum are from proprioceptive sources; this is particularly true of those travelling in the spino-cerebellar tracts and via the external cuneate nucleus. However, some impulses generated by exteroceptive stimuli also travel by these routes, although the principal pathway for these is through the anterolateral white columns of the cord and the nucleus of the lateral funiculus. Descending afferents to this latter ensure representation of face and head. Tecto-cerebellar connections, originating in the superior and inferior colliculi, are responsible for cerebellar representation of visual and auditory information respectively.

It has been shown that there are two areas of somatotopic representation in the cerebellar cortex, dependent on the exteroceptive input described above. The first of these is in the vermal and paravermal (intermediate) zones of the anterior lobe; here the body image lies on its back, head caudally, with the trunk representation in the vermis and the lower limbs in the paravermal zone; in man, the extremities of the upper limbs are functionally represented in the lateral lobes of the cerebellum. The second somatotopic area is in the paravermal zone (only) of the posterior part of the posterior lobe; there it is represented by two half-body images, with the head directed rostrally and the back lying against the vermis. In the rostralmost part of the posterior lobe (vermal and paravermal zones) are found two visual and two auditory receiving areas.

It is interesting that the anterior lobe tactile area is connected, by way of (cerebral) cortico-ponto-cerebellar fibres with the first somatic sensory area of the cerebral cortex, while the posterior lobe areas are similarly linked with the second somatic sensory cerebral area. Functionally, too, the cerebellar areas reflect the properties of SI and SII respectively. In general, it would appear as though exteroceptively-generated impulses impress images of the body pattern on the cerebellar cortex to serve as a spatial guide for cerebellar handling of rather diffusely-organized proprioceptive information.

It has already been mentioned that the cerebellar cortex projects on the deep nuclei in orderly fashion. This projection is organized not only in a mediolateral direction, from each of the three zones (vermal, paravermal and lateral) to each of the three nuclear groups (fastigial, interposed and dentate), but also in a rostrocaudal direction. It remains now to describe the efferent connections of the nuclei.

The axons of the dentate and interposed (emboliform and globose) nuclei leave the cerebellum exclusively by way of the brachium conjunctivum (Fig. 50). When these fibres reach the midbrain, they decussate completely (decussation of brachium conjunctivum) and come to ensheath the **red nucleus** (Fig. 27). Many of the axons terminate in the red nucleus; those that do not do so ascend further to the **thalamus** where they end in the **ventrolateral nucleus** (Fig. 46). Thence by a further relay this thalamic nucleus projects somatotopically to the motor cortex, i.e. the cortical areas of origin of the pyramidal and extrapyramidal motor systems (Fig. 47).

Immediately rostral to the decussation of the brachium conjunctivum, some (but by no means all) fibres bifurcate, and while one branch passes rostralward to establish the connections indicated in the previous paragraph, the other branches pass down into the medulla as the **descending limb of the brachium conjunctivum** (Fig. 50). These fibres establish connection with the **ventromedial reticular nuclei** of the pons and medulla (medial medullary motor reticular centres) and with the **nucleus of the facial nerve** (VII).

The efferent connections of the fastigial nuclei are a little more complicated. Most fastigial efferents reach the medulla oblongata by passing down in the inferior peduncle. About half of the fibres descend homolaterally as the **direct fastigiobulbar tract**. Many others cross to the other side of the cerebellum, hook round the intracerebellar part of the contralateral brachium conjunctivum, and then descend in to the medulla via the inferior peduncle of the side opposite to their origin. These indirect fastigiobulbar fibres are known as the **hook bundle** (uncinate fasciculus of Russell). Both the direct fastigiobulbar fibres and the hook bundle are distributed to the **vestibulbar nuclei** and the **dorsolateral reticular nuclei** of the pons and medulla (lateral medullary motor reticular centres) (Fig. 50).

The remaining efferent fibres from the fastigial nucleus decussate in the cerebellum and join the opposite superior peduncle as the accessory brachium conjunctivum (not shown in Fig. 50). These fibres do not decussate in the midbrain, as do the dentate and interposed efferents, but pass on up to the ventrolateral thalamic nucleus.

Before discussing cerebellar function in terms of its anatomy, it would be well to tabulate the composition of the peduncles:

1. Superior Peduncle.
   (a) Efferent: All fibres from dentate and interposed nuclei (brachium conjunctivum).
   Some fibres from contralateral fastigial nucleus (accessory brachium conjunctivum).
   (b) Afferent: Ventral spinocerebellar tract.
2. Middle Peduncle.
   Afferent: Pontocerebellar fibres.
3. Inferior Peduncle.
   (a) Efferent: Direct and indirect fastigiobulbar fibres.
   Corticovestibular fibres from flocculonodular lobe.
   (b) Afferent: Dorsal spino-cerebellar tract.
   Fibres from the external cuneate nucleus.
   Olivo-cerebellar fibres.
   Fibres from nucleus of lateral funiculus.
   Primary and secondary vestibular fibres.

Fibres from the paramedian reticular and peri-hypoglossal nuclei.

Functionally, it may be said that the cerebellum is a feedback mechanism whose purpose is to control movement while that movement is taking place. This occurs in both pyramidal and extrapyramidal systems, and is illustrated in simplified diagrammatic form in Fig. 52. When an impulse is initiated in the motor cerebral cortex which will eventually reach striated muscle, that cortex at the same time alerts the cerebellum via the pontine nuclei or the olive; thus the cerebellum is able to exert 'pre-control' over the movement which is about to take place. As soon as muscular movement actually occurs, proprioceptive impulses are conducted (more rapidly than any others in the neuraxis) via the spinocerebellar tracts or external cuneate nucleus to the cerebellar cortex.

The either/or fashion in which the cerebellum acts may be seen with reference to Fig. 51. All afferent input to the cerebellum (whether by **climbing fibres** from the olive or **mossy fibres** from other sources) is excitatory to cells of both the cerebellar nuclei and cortex; granule cells in the cerebellar cortex are also excitatory, as are the neurones of the deep nuclei. The Purkinje cells (which project to the cerebellar nuclei and lateral vestibular nucleus), the basket cells, and all other cortical interneurones are inhibitory. Remembering that the rich interconnections of the cerebellar cortex allows impulses to travel by a number of alternative pathways, it can be seen that afferent impulses may excite Purkinje cells, either directly (climbing fibres) or via granule cells (mossy fibres); this will cause the Purkinje cells to send inhibitory impulses to the nuclear cells, thus cancelling out excitatory influences arriving by other pathways ('disfacilitation'), and so having a null net effect on the output of the nuclear cell onto upper motor neurones (rubrospinal or reticulospinal) or VL cells projecting to motor cortex (left-hand side of Fig. 51). An alternative pathway (right-hand side of Fig. 51) would allow afferent impulses to excite inhibitory interneurones which prevent Purkinje cells from inhibiting the nuclear cells to which they project; this allows excitatory impulses to fire the nuclear cells and thus

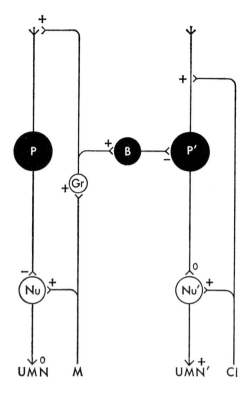

FIG. 51. Highly schematized diagram of cerebellar mechanisms. Excitatory input by either mossy (M) or climbing (Cl) fibres acts on cerebellar nuclear neurone (Nu) and granule (Gr) or Purkinje (P) cell. Granule cell may excite Purkinje cell, causing it to fire and inhibit nuclear cell giving a net zero effect on upper motor neurone (UMN) or VL cell which it innervates. On right of diagram, granule cell is shown exciting inhibitory basket cell (B), which prevents Purkinje cell (P') from inhibiting nuclear cell Nu', giving a net facilitatory effect to upper motor neurone UMN'. Due to interconnections and depending on input patterns, the effect of any one nuclear cell on the neurones to which it projects may be either o or +.

facilitate the neurones to which they in turn project. It is important to realize that the pathways to be followed by impulses, and therefore the form of output, are dependent on the pattern of afferent input; therefore the effect on any one neurone to which the cerebellar nuclei project may be either zero or facilitation. In accordance with the pattern of its input from motor centres and proprioceptors, the final integrated output of the cerebellum serves to raise the level of excitability of the upper motor neurones (some

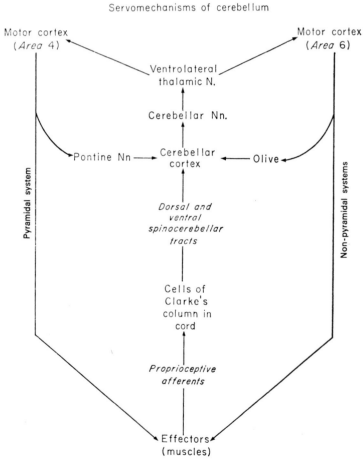

FIG. 52. Diagram to illustrate cerebellar servomechanisms (explanations in text).

of which may have an inhibitory effect on lower motor neurones) appropriate for the movement in question.

It is known that the cerebellum is able to influence reticulo-spinal neurones which control both α and γ motoneurones. Although, in cerebellar disease, the disorder of movement is more dramatic, it must be remembered that cerebellar control also influences tone.

Because the cerebellum 'feeds' on proprioceptive information, cerebellar lesions chiefly declare themselves during movement, when they produce 'intention tremor'. For the same reason, there is no tremor at rest in cerebellar disease.

CHAPTER FIFTEEN

The Rhinencephalon
and Hypothalamus

The rhinencephalon is phylogenetically the oldest part of the fore-brain, and its anatomy is complicated only because it has been pushed out of the way and overgrown by more recently developed parts. The word means 'smellbrain', and it was formerly thought to be concerned only with the sensation of smell. Comparative studies, however, show that the rhinencephalon is virtually the only representative of the telencephalon in certain lowly creatures; and they certainly do a great deal more than smell (in the purely sensory meaning of the word). The hypothalamus is also a very ancient part of the brain, which is structurally and functionally intimately tied up with the rhinencephalon. In general, it may be said that much is known about the anatomical connections of the rhinencephalon, but little about its functions, while a great deal is known about the physiology of the hypothalamus, but little of the anatomical pathways by which these functions are subserved.

When the olfactory nerves pass through the cribriform plate of the ethmoid bone, they pass straight into the **olfactory bulb,** in which they terminate. Secondary olfactory neurones run back-wards in the **olfactory tract,** clearly visible on the orbital surface of the frontal lobe. Just in front of the **anterior perforated substance,** the olfactory tract splits into **medial** and **lateral olfactory striae.** While it is impossible to illustrate the further course of the lateral stria on the two planes of paper, careful examination of the base of an actual brain will show that it runs up into the lower part of the **frontal operculum,** where it becomes blended with the cortex. Thence the cortex of the rhinencephalon can be traced as an uninterrupted band across the **limen insulae** into the **uncus** and **hippocampal gyrus** (Fig. 39). The rhinencephalic part of the frontal operculum is known as **prepyriform** cortex while the limen insulae and uncus constitute the **intermediate pyriform cortex**. The hippocampal gyrus itself forms the **entorhinal cortex**.

Physiological experiments have shown that the prepyriform and intermediate pyriform cortices are directly associated with the sense of smell, i.e. olfactory sensations are evoked when they are electrically stimulated. But this is not the case with the entorhinal cortex, which should be regarded as an olfactory association area. Thus only those parts of the rhinencephalon so far described are concerned with the conscious sense of smell. The system is remarkable in that it runs by a chain of neurones from sense organ to cortex without relaying through the thalamus; phylogenetically, the thalamus was developed after the rhinencephalon.

The **hippocampus**, as can be seen in coronal section (Fig. 53), represents an inrolling from the hippocampal gyrus. It is a primitive kind of motor cortex, in which large pyramidal cells predominate. The axons from these cells appear on the upper surface of the hippocampus as the **fimbria**, and, turning at a right angle, run upward as the posterior column of the **fornix** (see Chapter 9). The course of the fornix has already been described, but in fact only about half of its fibres end in the mammillary body of the hypothalamus, in which its anterior columns appear macroscopically to terminate. The other connections of the fornix will be described with reference to Fig. 54, in which all the important connections of the rhinencephalon are set out in diagrammatic form. Axons from the body of the fornix turn down to enter directly the medial part of the **hypothalamus**; as the body turns down to become the anterior columns, further fibres are detached to join the **septal area**. This is the name given to the grey matter just in front of the lamina terminalis on the medial surface of the frontal lobe (Fig. 28). Finally, as the anterior column of the fornix bends back towards the mammillary body, many fibres by-pass this destination in order to pass directly to (i) the anterior and intralaminar nuclei of the thalamus, and (ii) the dorsal tegmental (descending reticular) nucleus of the midbrain. The mammillary nuclei themselves project by secondary fibres to both the anterior thalamic and midbrain descending reticular nuclei; to the first by means of the **mammillothalamic tract,** passing almost directly upwards, and to the second by means of the **mammillotegmental tract,** passing caudally.

The anterior thalamic nuclei project point-to-point on to the **cingulate gyrus,** which lies above the corpus callosum. Stretched over the top of the corpus callosum, running in an antero-posterior direction (i.e. at right angles to the callosal fibres) and hidden in the callosal sulcus, are three fibre-bands, called the **medial** and **lateral longitudinal striae,** and the **cingulum.** By means of

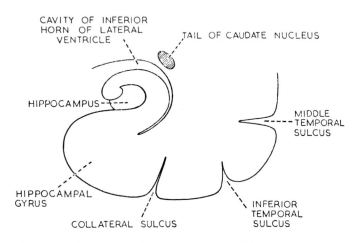

FIG. 53. Coronal section through the right temporal lobe, viewed from behind, to show how the hippocampus is inrolled from the hippocampal gyrus.

these, impulses from the cingulate gyrus are able to reach the hippocampus, and so the circuit is completed (see Fig. 54).

Those fibres of the lateral olfactory stria that do not terminate in the prepyriform cortex run into the **amygdaloid nucleus** (Figs. 33 and 34), in the floor of the temporal pole (Chapter 9). It will be remembered that the amygdaloid nucleus is joined by the tail of the caudate nucleus. The efferent discharge pathway from the amygdaloid nucleus is called the **stria terminalis,** and accompanies the caudate nucleus, but in reverse direction. From the dorsal aspect, the fibres of the stria terminalis may be seen in the groove between the thalamus and the body and head of the caudate nucleus (usually accompanied by one or more prominent veins). When the stria terminalis reaches the medial side of the head of the caudate, it ends in the **septal nuclei** (area).

Apart from the fornix and stria terminalis, the septal nuclei also receive fibres from the **medial olfactory stria**. Some of these fibres are direct, and some are interrupted by scattered grey cells which lie in the anterior perforated substance. In lower animals this cell group is bigger, and is dignified with the name of **olfactory tubercle**; the appellation of this sub-primate prominence is frequently transferred to the corresponding depression in man. Those fibres of the medial olfactory stria which do not pass to the septal nuclei cross in the **anterior commissure** to the olfactory bulb of the other side (Fig. 54).

The septal nuclei discharge their efferent impulses by two pathways. One is the **medial forebrain bundle**, which leads directly to (and from) the hypothalamus. More will be said of this later in the present chapter. The other is the **stria medullaris** (Chapter 9), which leads back along the dorsomedial border of the thalamus to the **habenular nuclei** (Fig. 29). These latter give off fibres which curve ventrocaudally through the midbrain as the **habenulo-interpeduncular tract** to reach the **interpeduncular nucleus**, which lies, as its name suggests, in the ventral fork of the midbrain, between the two cerebral peduncles. Further fibres from the interpeduncular nucleus discharge caudally, joining with efferents from the dorsal tegmental nucleus to reach those same lower motor reticular centres as are utilized by the 'extrapyramidal' motor system.

Thus the rhinencephalon discharges by two routes, the dorsal tegmental and interpeduncular nuclei, into the nonpyramidal motor pathways which will eventually affect skeletal muscle; and by three ways into the hypothalamus: by the medial forebrain bundle from the septal nuclei, by fibres from the body of the fornix into the dorsomedial hypothalamus, and by the anterior columns of the fornix into the mammillary nuclei (bodies).

Macroscopically, the uncus and hippocampal gyrus, together with the hippocampus, fornix, and cingulate gyrus (which is

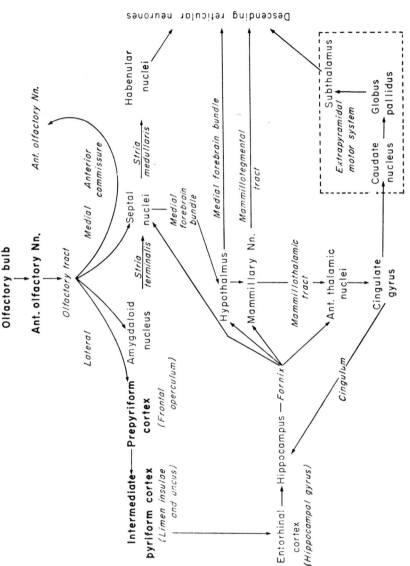

FIG. 54. Diagram to show the connections of the rhinencephalon. Only the structures in bold type

continuous around the splenium of the corpus callosum with the hippocampal gyrus) form a belt (limbus) around the corpus callosum which is known as the **limbic lobe**: it is virtually co-extensive with the rhinencephalon.

The gross anatomy of the hypothalamus, in the wall of the third ventricle below and in front of the thalamus, has already been explained (Chapter 8). Its anterior limit is the optic chiasma, its posterior the mammillary bodies. In a coronal section through the middle part of the hypothalamus (Fig. 55), it may be seen that the anterior (descending) column of the fornix divides the hypo-thalamus into a lateral and a medial part. The **lateral hypothal-amus** consists of scattered cells through which run the fibres of the medial forebrain bundle. The medial hypothalamus (Fig. 56) consists of a fairly large group of nuclei, not all of which need be remembered.

Most anteriorly, above the chiasma, and rostral to the hypo-thalamus proper, lies the **pre-optic region**. Behind this in the medial hypothalamus lie the **supra-optic** and **paraventricular** nuclei, whose efferent fibres pass as the **supra-optico-hypo-physeal** tract to the posterior pituitary gland (pars nervosa). Immediately caudal to these the medial hypothalamus consists of the upper part of the pituitary stalk, known as the **tuberal region**; this contains the dorsomedial, ventromedial, posterior hypo-thalamic, and tuberal nuclei. It is the dorsomedial nucleus which chiefly receives those hippocampal efferent fibres which detach themselves from the body of the fornix. Below the tuberal region is the infundibulum.

Most posteriorly in the medial hypothalamus is the **mammil-lary group** of nuclei, the medial of which receives the anterior column of the fornix (from the hippocampus). The mammillary nuclei discharge (a) via the **mammillotegmental** tract to descending midbrain reticular neurones, and thence to lower motor reticular centres, and (b) via the **mammillo-thalamic** tract to the anterior thalamic group of nuclei, and thence, in a point-to-point fashion to the transitional cortex (allocortex) of the cingulate gyrus.

Cells in various parts of the hypothalamus may be stimulated

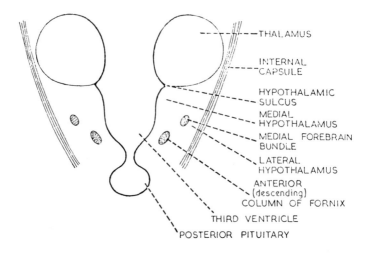

FIG. 55. Diagrammatic coronal section through the diencephalon to show the medial and lateral parts of the hypothalamus, and their relations.

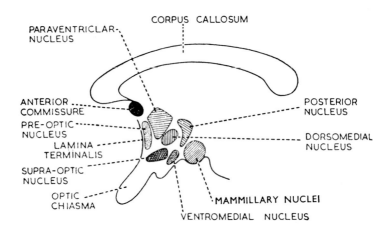

FIG. 56. Nuclei of the medial hypothalamus projected on to a medial sagittal section of the diencephalon (after Le Gros Clark).

(or inhibited) in two ways, nervous or physico-chemical. The nervous connections to the hypothalamus are:

(i) The medial forebrain bundle, which runs from the septal (rhinencephalic) nuclei anteriorly to the mesencephalic tegmentum caudally (Fig. 55). This affords two-way connections (ascending and descending) between the regions mentioned, plus the (lateral) pre-optic nuclei.

(ii) The fornix, bringing afferent impulses from the (rhinencephalic) hippocampus.

(iii) Fibres from the rhinencephalic amygdaloid complex to the ventromedial hypothalamic nucleus.

(iv) Cortical afferents from orbito-frontal regions of the regions of the neocortex—which in their turn receive a point-to-point projection from the dorsomedial nucleus of the thalamus (Chapter 12).

(v) Ascending afferents to the hypothalamus enter from the midbrain tegmentum in the medial forebrain bundle and the **mammillary peduncle**. The midbrain reticular regions which project into the hypothalamus receive ascending visceral afferent impulses, some of which have come up from the spinal cord, and probably relay in the caudal part of the solitary nucleus and again in the lower brainstem reticular formation before reaching midbrain reticular centres, as well as somatically-generated information.

In addition to these purely nervous afferent connections, cells in various parts of the hypothalamus may be directly affected by the physical or chemical properties of the blood in which they are bathed. In this connection, it should be noted that the hypothalamus, in spite of its phylogenetic antiquity, has a far higher capillary density than any other part of the brain (see Chapter 16). Specific sensitivity to the following has been established:

(a) Osmotic pressure—supraoptic and paraventricular nuclei.

(b) Temperature—the anterior part of the hypothalamus reacts to high blood temperature, and the posterior part to low.

Other hypothalamic cells are sensitive to the level of various hormones and substances such as glucose and sodium chloride in the blood.

The overall function of the hypothalamus is clear. It is the centre exercising control over the internal milieu of the organism; and if the physico-chemical conditions of the body are not maintained within narrow limits, life rapidly ceases. How this is done may now be briefly described.

In fact, the centres concerned with tonic control and reflex adjustment of cardiac and respiratory activity are in the lower brainstem reticular formation, and are quite capable of functioning normally when cut off from all hypothalamic influence. The inspiratory and vasopressor 'centres' are a part of the facilitatory descending reticular system, and the expiratory and vasodilator centres of the inhibitory descending reticular system.

The hypothalamus is concerned, as befits a higher centre, with integrated reactions to particular situations. The following functions may be attributed to various parts of the hypothalamus:

(i) Anterior hypothalamus (including pre-optic regions)
    (a) Bladder control (medial pre-optic region)
    (b) Heat loss (anterior hypothalamus)
    (c) Somnolence (pre-optic region)
(ii) Middle hypothalamus
    (a) Appetite (level of ventromedial nucleus)
    (b) Thirst (dorsolateral to supra-optic nucleus)
(iii) Posterior hypothalamus
    (a) Heat retention
    (b) Sexual behaviour
    (c) Wakefulness.

Three comments should be made upon the above table. First, the hypothalamus is not the only cerebral structure concerned with sleep and wakefulness; other parts of the (ascending) reticular arousal system and telencephalon should also be taken into account. Secondly, only the pre-optic region is concerned with purely parasympathetic autonomic activity; gut motility as well as bladder contraction can be evoked by stimulation of these regions. All autonomic activity evoked from the hypothalamus proper can be explained on the basis of facilitation or inhibition of sympathetic activity. Thirdly, it should be noted that every single one of the activities attributed to the hypothalamus proper involves the activity of striated muscle as well as of smooth muscle and glands; the brain does not make the clear contradistinction between 'somatic' and 'visceral' which some teachers do.

The efferent discharge pathways by which the hypothalamus brings about these effects are:

(i) The descending fibres of the medial forebrain bundle.

(ii) The mammillo-tegmental tract.

(iii) The **dorsal longitudinal fasciculus**, which arises in the medial hypothalamus rostral to the mammillary region.

All these three pathways discharge into the descending reticular system by way of synapses in the midbrain tegmentum. For the sake of completeness, we may here enumerate two further efferent projections from the hypothalamus, which are probably more concerned with hypothalamorhinencephalic function:

(iv) The mammillo-thalamic tract.

(v) **Periventricular fibres,** which pass up in the wall of the third ventricle from the hypothalamus to the midline (periventricular) and dorsomedial nuclei of the thalamus.

Just as the hypothalamus is directly affected by physico-chemical factors, so is it intimately concerned with endocrine output. Its humoral activity may be conveniently divided into posterior and anterior pituitary functions:

The fibres of the supra-optico hypophyseal tract end in relationship with the capillary bed of the posterior pituitary (neurohypophysis), in between the pituicyte cells, which are derived from neuroglia. The terminals of these neurones, whose cell bodies lie in the supra-optic and paraventricular nuclei, instead of liberating a transmitter substance onto effectors or other neurones, secrete **antidiuretic hormone** directly into the blood stream; this substance passes in the circulation to the kidneys, where it has the effect of increasing tubular reabsorption of water. Thus lesions of the supra-optico-hypophyseal tract or its cells of origin cause **diabetes insipidus**, through failure to reabsorb water. The hormone is secreted (or not) in direct response to the osmotic pressure of the blood bathing the supra-optic and paraventricular cells.

A second substance liberated by the terminals of the supra-optico-hypophyseal tract in lactating females is the **galactogenic**

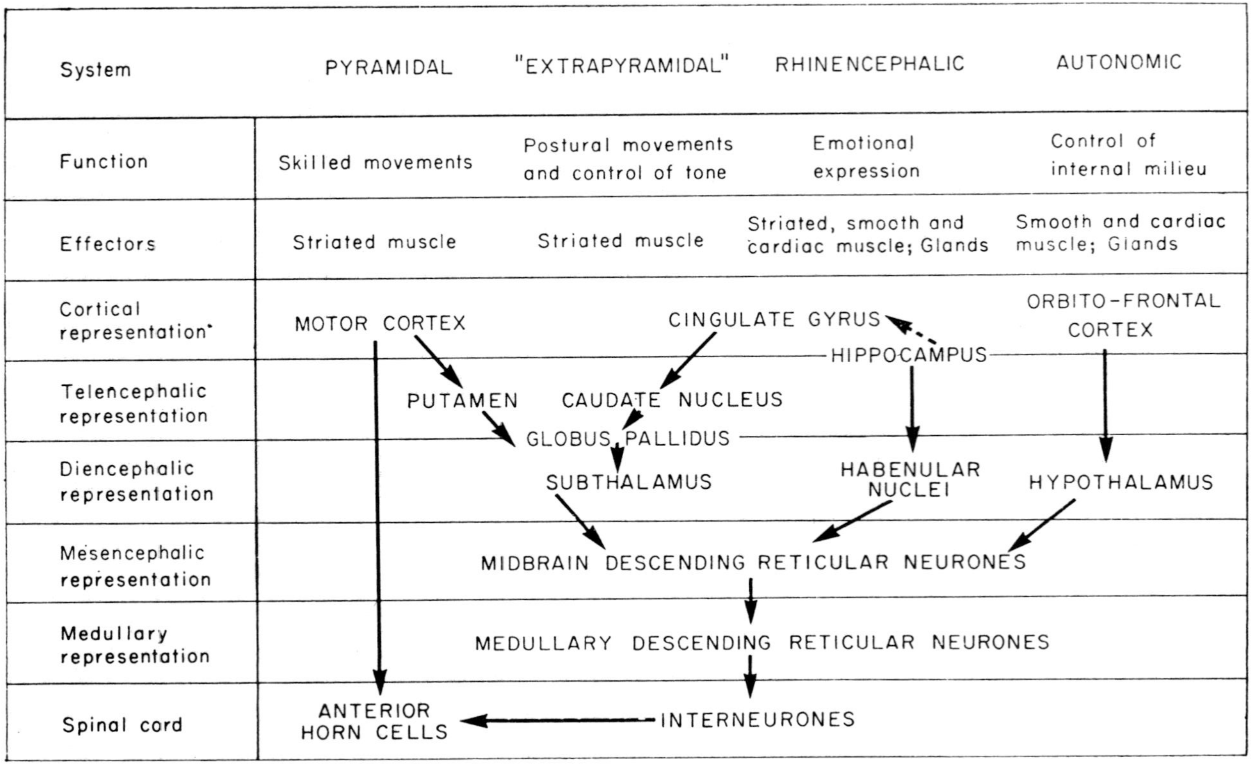

System	PYRAMIDAL	"EXTRAPYRAMIDAL"	RHINENCEPHALIC	AUTONOMIC
Function	Skilled movements	Postural movements and control of tone	Emotional expression	Control of internal milieu
Effectors	Striated muscle	Striated muscle	Striated, smooth and cardiac muscle; Glands	Smooth and cardiac muscle; Glands
Cortical representation*	MOTOR CORTEX		CINGULATE GYRUS — HIPPOCAMPUS	ORBITO-FRONTAL CORTEX
Telencephalic representation		PUTAMEN CAUDATE NUCLEUS GLOBUS PALLIDUS		
Diencephalic representation		SUBTHALAMUS	HABENULAR NUCLEI	HYPOTHALAMUS
Mesencephalic representation	MIDBRAIN DESCENDING RETICULAR NEURONES			
Medullary representation	MEDULLARY DESCENDING RETICULAR NEURONES			
Spinal cord	ANTERIOR HORN CELLS — INTERNEURONES			

FIG. 57. Diagram to show the functions, connections, and inter-relations of the motor-pathways. The only feedback circuit shown in this diagram is from the hippocampus to the cortex of the cingulate gyrus (broken line).

hormone, which (humorally) stimulates milk secretion and ejection. The afferent side of this reflex is purely neural, and arises from peripheral fibres in the nipple in response to suckling. Hypothalamic control of the anterior pituitary is more remote, but just as effective. The hypothalamic efferent nerve fibres concerned end in association with capillaries in the median eminence of the pituitary stalk. These capillaries form one end of the **hypophyseal portal system**, the other being in the anterior pituitary (adenohypophysis). Thus substances secreted into the capillaries by nerve terminals pass in the blood to the anterior pituitary, where they bring about various effects, including the secretion of thyrotrophic, adrenocorticotrophic, and gonadotrophic hormones into the systemic blood stream by the anterior pituitary cells.

It may be noted that there is nothing magic or peculiar about this process of **neurosecretion**. It differs from the liberation of transmitter substance at a synapse only in that in neurosecretion the transmitter substance is not immediately destroyed by an enzyme, and acts at a distance via the bloodstream instead of locally on a postsynaptic membrane. There is evidence to suggest that in some instances the same substance may act at some sites as a synaptic transmitter and at others as a neurosecretion (neurohormone). Furthermore, it now appears probable that neurosecretion may also occur (though to a much lesser degree) at some brain sites other than the hypothalamus.

The functions of the non-olfactory part of the rhinencephalon, being connected as it is both with the hypothalamus and with skeletal motor systems, is a little more difficult to understand. It has been pointed out that although man is a microsmatic animal, i.e. he depends only very slightly on his sense of smell, he has, both absolutely and relatively, the largest hippocampus in the animal kingdom.

The rhinencephalon appears to be responsible for emotion or **affect**; and its motor discharges, linked with those of the hypothalamus, for emotional expression. It is known, for example, that a balance between amygdaloid complex, hypothalamus, and cingulate gyrus (limbic cortex) are responsible for the manifestation of rage and docility. Hippocampal projections, via the fornix, to the intralaminar nuclei of the thalamus may be responsible for the changes in muscle tone which accompany emotional states ('tense with rage' or 'weak with laughter'); for it will be recalled that the intralaminar nuclei project to the putamen and caudate nucleus, which are parts of the 'extrapyramidal' motor system controlling muscle tone.

Emotional expression involves autonomic changes, such as pilo-erection (goose-flesh), blood pressure changes, etc., as well as skeletal muscular movements; these latter are particularly seen in the face, which would call for a particularly large rhinencephalic influence on the seventh cranial nerve motor nucleus. While the known rhinencephalic connections are well suited to the functions which are attributed to it, it may be helpful to recall that olfactory sensations, more than those of any other modality, evoke emotional responses, however fleetingly.

The close anatomical and functional association between rhin-encephalon and hypothalamus is to be explained by the fact that primitive vertebrates depend primarily on the chemical sense (i.e. olfaction) to find their food and their mates—in other words to ensure the survival of the individual and of the species. Higher vertebrates, including man, sometimes manage to put their emotional drive to other uses.

The primacy of rhinencephalic effect is seen in the result of bilateral ablation of the hippocampus: this causes inability of the neocortex to retain new information—i.e. to learn and to remember; but to acquire new information depends on motivation, so that the first phase of memory formation may be said to be an emotional rather than a rational act. The analogy may be made that the neocortex is like a computer, which is indiscriminately fed with all sorts of information by afferent systems through the thalamus; but that this vast and intricate computer is programmed by the rhinencephalon.

There is a close functional integration between all motor systems, and this is paralleled by an anatomical integration which is illustrated in Fig. 57.

CHAPTER SIXTEEN

The Blood Supply of the Central Nervous System

Although the brain only accounts for 2 per cent of the body weight, it receives 16·6 per cent of the total cardiac output and consumes 20 per cent of the oxygen used by the whole body. Nerve cells can only live for a few minutes without oxygen. Within the nervous system, there are considerable quantitative differences in the blood supply of various regions. In particular, the capillary density of the grey matter is very much higher than that of the white matter; and average blood flow through grey matter is thrice that through white. Within the grey matter itself, there are differences which usually vary directly with the phylogenetic age, with the notable exception of the hypothalamus (see preceding chapter). Thus the hippocampus and globus pallidus, for example, being very ancient parts of the brain, have a very much less rich blood supply than the more recently developed caudate nucleus and putamen; the cortices of the cerebrum and cerebellum, being of the most recent origin, have the richest blood supply of all.

The principles governing the arterial supply to the central nervous system are simple and straightforward. Essentially, there is a longitudinal ventral arterial trunk (Fig. 58), which gives off two kinds of branch: circular (**coronal**), which encircles and supplies the periphery of the neuraxis, and deep, which penetrate the nervous substance from the ventral aspect. While the branches of adjacent circular arteries make more or less tenuous anastomoses with one another, there is, at least from a functional point of view, no anastomosis between deep branches. The longitudinal ventral arterial trunk is fed at various levels by extraneuraxial vessels.

The basic plan is seen at its most typical in the spinal cord. The longitudinal trunk is the **anterior spinal artery**, which runs between the lips of the anterior (ventral) median fissure. It is fed asymmetrically (unilaterally) by arteries which enter through the intervertebral foramina; there are usually two in the cervical region, three in the thoracic, and two in the lumbar spine. The most constant of these feeders is the artery of Adamkiewicz which enters through the second left lumbar interspace. At its top (rostral) end, the anterior spinal artery is fed (classically formed) bilaterally and symmetrically from the unequal bifurcation of the **vertebral artery** on each side.

The deep branches of the anterior spinal artery are called **sulcal** branches, because they pass up the anterior median sulcus to penetrate into the spinal grey matter (Fig. 58). Each sulcal artery supplies the grey matter on either the left *or* the right side of the spinal cord, but not both. Moreover, successive sulcal branches do not necessarily alternate. The coronal branches pass round the external surface of the spinal cord, giving off branches which supply the white matter and the tips of the dorsal horns of the grey matter. Longitudinal branches of the coronal branches anastomose somewhat irregularly along the lines of the dorsal roots on each side, to form discontinuous **posterior spinal arteries**.

There is in fact an interruption in the visible continuity of the ventral arterial trunk at the level of the pyramidal decussation. Rostrally, the median longitudinal vessel continues as the **basilar artery** (Figs. 58, 59), which appears to be formed by the major terminal branches of its bilaterally symmetrical feeders, the vertebral arteries. In this lower brainstem region, great expansion of some coronal branches can already be seen, in order to supply the cerebellum on the dorsal aspect of the brainstem. Thus the highly-convoluted **posterior inferior cerebellar arteries** (Fig. 58) (which in fact arise from the vertebral arteries before they join the basilar artery) supply not only the lateral aspect of the medulla oblongata but also much of the caudal cerebellum as well as the choroid plexus of the fourth ventricle. Two similar coronal branches arise from the basilar artery, the **anterior inferior** and **superior cerebellar arteries**. Between these named coronal branches which extend to supply the cerebellum may be seen

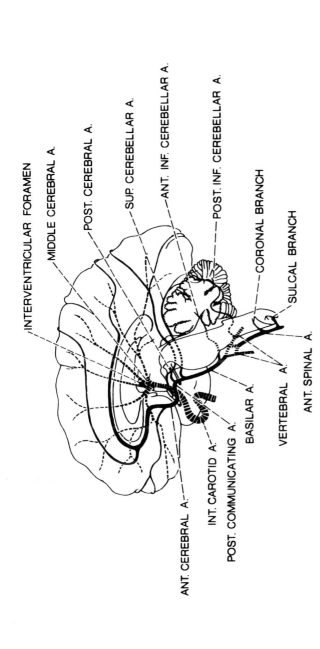

INTERVENTRICULAR FORAMEN

MIDDLE CEREBRAL A.

POST. CEREBRAL A.

SUP. CEREBELLAR A.

ANT. INF. CEREBELLAR A.

POST. INF. CEREBELLAR A.

CORONAL BRANCH

SULCAL BRANCH

ANT. SPINAL A.

VERTEBRAL A.

BASILAR A.

POST. COMMUNICATING A.

INT. CAROTID A.

ANT. CEREBRAL A.

FIG. 58. The arterial system of the neuraxis viewed from the side. The ventral longitudinal arterial trunk is made up successively of the anterior spinal, basilar, posterior communicating, and anterior cerebral arteries, reinforced by the paired vertebral and internal carotid arteries. Enlarged and named coronal branches are shown in interrupted lines when they are on the lateral side of the brain.

unnamed ordinary coronal branches encircling the lower brain-stem, thus restoring one's faith in the orderly arrangement of the neuraxial blood supply.

At its rostral end in the interpeduncular fossa, the basilar artery gives off two pairs of enlarged coronal branches, both of which wind round the midbrain. The caudalmore of these, the superior cerebellar artery, has already been mentioned; after reaching the dorsal aspect of the midbrain, it expands to supply the superior surface of the rostral part of the cerebellum. The rostralmore pair of coronal arteries, separated at their origins from the superior cerebellars by the emergence of the third nerve, are the **posterior cerebral arteries** (Fig. 58). After winding round the midbrain, they pass under the splenium of the corpus callosum, supplying it and giving off a posterior choroidal artery which passes forward beneath the splenium to the choroid plexuses of the third and lateral ventricles. The major part of the posterior cerebral artery is swept backwards along the medial surface of the posterior (occipital) lobe of the cerebral hemisphere on each side. The principal branch occupies the calcarine fissure, thus ensuring the arterial supply of the primary visual area of the cortex.

At the point in the interpeduncular fossa where the two posterior cerebral arteries are given off (classically known as the bifurcation of the basilar artery), numerous deep branches penetrate the brain substance just behind the mammillary bodies, when these arteries are pulled out (with the basilar artery from which they arise), the floor of the interpeduncular fossa is left looking like a pepper pot, and is here known as the **posterior perforated substance** (Fig. 59).

Because the forebrain is divided into two cerebral hemispheres, the principle of a ventral arterial trunk with coronal and deep branches becomes bilateral at this level. Continuing forward from the bifurcation of the basilar artery, i.e. from the roots of the posterior cerebral arteries, the **posterior communicating artery** (Fig. 58) passes across the floor of the diencephalon on each side, until by the side of the optic chiasm it is joined by its enormous

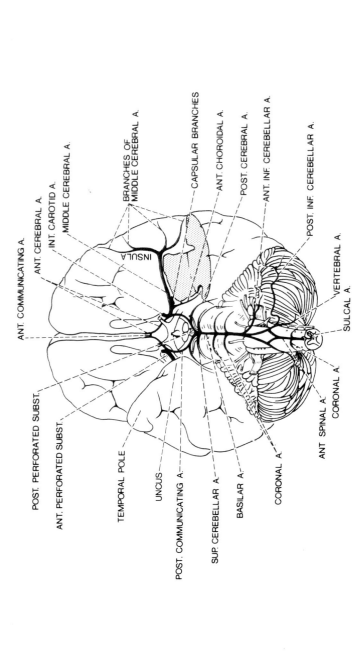

ANT. COMMUNICATING A.

ANT. CEREBRAL A.

INT. CAROTID A.

MIDDLE CEREBRAL A.

BRANCHES OF
MIDDLE CEREBRAL A.

CAPSULAR BRANCHES

ANT. CHOROIDAL A.

POST. CEREBRAL A.

ANT. INF. CEREBELLAR A.

POST. INF. CEREBELLAR A.

VERTEBRAL A.

SULCAL A.

INSULA

POST. PERFORATED SUBST.

ANT. PERFORATED SUBST.

TEMPORAL POLE

UNCUS

POST. COMMUNICATING A.

SUP. CEREBELLAR A.

BASILAR A.

CORONAL A.

CORONAL A.

ANT. SPINAL A.

FIG. 59. The arterial system of the neuraxis viewed from the ventral aspect. The temporal pole and the operculae of the left hemisphere have been removed in order to reveal the course of the middle cerebral artery.

feeder, the **internal carotid artery*** (Figs. 58, 59). In fact the posterior communicating artery, although it is technically part of the ventral arterial trunk of the forebrain, looks like a miserable little strand of arterial tissue joining the internal carotid/middle cerebral artery and the basilar/posterior cerebral artery—hence its name. At the point where the internal carotid joins the posterior communicating artery, there is given off the largest coronal branch of the whole cerebral arterial system, the **middle cerebral artery** (Fig. 59). It is classically described as one of the two terminal branches of the internal carotid artery, and it is frequently the beginning of the middle cerebral artery, rather than the internal carotid itself, with which the posterior communicating artery actually communicates.

The course of the middle cerebral artery lies on the axis of growth of the forebrain (Fig. 58)—the transverse line running through the interventricular foramina to emerge from the lips of the lateral fissure after passing through the insula of each side (Chapter 9, Fig. 31). From its origin lateral to the optic chiasm, the middle cerebral artery runs out laterally in the stem of the lateral fissure—i.e. above the temporal pole (Fig. 59)—until it reaches the insula, where it breaks up into branches. These turn upward on the surface of the insula, then down again on the inner surface of the frontal and parietal opercula to emerge from the lips of the lateral fissure whence they spread out to cover and supply most of the lateral aspect of the hemisphere. This includes, functionally, the whole of the primary auditory area and its associative region, the motor and sensory speech areas, and the primary motor and somatic sensory representations from the head to the hip joint. The apparently complex course of the middle cerebral artery over the insula and opercula are of course explained by the way the forebrain grows. As the middle cerebral artery enters the stem of the lateral fissure, it gives off:

(a) a backward-running **anterior choroidal** branch which rolls

---

* It should be noted that the blood supply of the dura mater comes from the *external* carotid artery, and not the *internal*, as does that of the brain.

into the inferior horn of the lateral ventricle with the hippocampus and supplies the choroid plexus; and

(b) a number of important deep branches which supply the internal capsule and lentiform nucleus (**lenticulostriate** branch) as well as the head of the caudate nucleus and part of the thalamus.

Returning to the ventral longitudinal arterial trunk of each hemisphere, rostral to the junction of the posterior communicating and internal carotid/middle cerebral arteries, it is continued forward as the **anterior cerebral artery** (Fig. 58) (classically considered as one of the two terminal branches of the internal carotid). From their origin at the side of the optic chiasm, the anterior cerebral arteries of the two sides run forwards and towards each other, dorsal to the optic nerves, and reach the under side of the rostrum of the corpus callosum, at which point they are very close together. They are here joined together by a midline anastomotic branch called the **anterior communicating artery** (Fig. 59). The initial portion of the anterior cerebral artery crosses the depression between the lateral and medial olfactory striae (Chapter 15), and at this point gives off its deep (perforating) branches, thus giving rise to an **anterior perforated substance** (Fig. 59) on each side. The parts of the two anterior cerebral arteries beyond the anterior communicating branch follow round the external border of the genu of the corpus callosum, to reach the dorsal aspect of the body as **pericallosal arteries** (Fig. 58), giving off coronal branches of which the chief runs in the cingulate sulcus. Thus both the anterior cerebral/pericallosal arteries representing the ventral median trunk, and its coronal branches, not being on the axis of the forebrain, are swept round in the direction of growth (Chapter 9; Fig. 31); they supply the medial surface and dorsomedial rim of the lateral surface of the hemisphere as far back as the parieto-occipital fissure, being thus responsible for the lower limb representation of the primary somato-sensory and motor areas, and the whole of the supplementary motor area.

The anterior communicating artery completes a ring of arteries on the ventral surface of the diencephalon, encircling the pituitary stalk and optic chiasm, and known as the **Circle of Willis** (Fig.

59). Classically it is considered to be formed by the initial segments of the posterior cerebral arteries following the bifurcation of the basilar artery, the posterior communicating arteries, the initial segments of the anterior cerebral arteries, and the single anterior communicating artery. Viewed thus, its inputs are considered to be the vertebro-basilar artery and the two internal carotids; and its outputs the three pairs of cerebral arteries.

It has long been known that the Circle of Willis, in health, is only a potential anastomosis, as is shown by cerebral angiography. When a radio-opaque medium is injected into a vertebral artery, only the branches of the vertebro-basilar system up to and including the posterior cerebral arteries are filled. Similarly, injection into an internal carotid artery fills only the cerebral arteries of the injected side; in 70% of cases only the anterior and middle cerebral arteries become radio-opaque, while in the remaining 30% the ipsilateral posterior cerebral artery also fills through the posterior communicating artery.

The Circle of Willis, which is rarely symmetrical, is thus a potential anastomosis, and may come into play if one of its constituents slowly (but not suddenly) becomes obliterated. However, the arterial circle has not, as maintained by some anthropocentric anatomists, been provided by a beneficent Providence against the senescent time when cerebral arteriosclerosis sets in. All vertebrates, the vast majority of whom do not live beyond what we would call middle age, have a Circle of Willis. Its probable importance is during the rapid embryonic growth of the brain; by ensuring an equal flow of oxygen and metabolites to the two sides, it guards against the possibility of asymmetric growth of the hemispheres.

The venous drainage of the spinal cord and brain shows the usual multiplicity of veins in comparison with arteries.

In the spinal cord, the sulcal veins drain both sides, not one like the arteries, and they are fewer in number, and not venae comitantes of the arteries. They drain into an **anterior spinal vein,** which ends in the vertebral veins, but which is also connected through each emergent nerve root with the **extradural vertebral venous sinuses,** and so through the intervertebral foramina with the vertebral veins in the neck, and azygos and hemiazygos in the thorax, and their tributaries, the ascending lumbar veins, in the abdomen. Thus all blood from the neuraxis drains eventually into the superior vena cava. For the importance of this, see Chapter 3.

There are also coronal veins and posterior spinal veins corresponding to the arteries, and in addition a posterior median septal vein. They are all connected with the leash-like plexuses surrounding the emergent nerve roots, and the longitudinal veins drain at their upper ends into the vertebral veins. The areas of drainage of these veins correspond to the arterial areas of supply.

The veins of the brain stem up to and including the posterior cerebral vein correspond to the arteries, draining into the basilar and vertebral vein, and it is unnecessary to give further explanation of them. But in the cerebral hemispheres, the venous drainage differs from the arterial supply in being served by two sets of vessels, a superficial and a deep. The superficial veins drain the cortex. The **superior cerebral veins** run into the superior sagittal sinus, opening into it against the direction of flow. The veins of the middle part of the cortex flow into the **superficial middle cerebral vein**, in the lateral fissure. At least one anastomotic vein (the vein of Trolard) joins the superficial middle cerebral vein to the superior sagittal sinus. The veins of the temporal lobe flow into the transverse and superficial petrosal sinuses. The transverse sinus is connected to the superficial middle cerebral vein by the anastomotic **vein of Labbé**; and the superficial middle cerebral vein itself opens into the cavernous sinus.

The deeper parts of the hemisphere drain into the **deep middle cerebral vein**, which also runs in the lateral fissure. The medial surface of the hemisphere is drained by the **anterior cerebral vein**, corresponding to the artery. The anterior and deep middle cerebral veins meet at the root of the lateral fissure and join to form the **basal vein**. This winds round the deepest part of the cerebral peduncles, in company with the optic tract, until it reaches a posterior position just under the splenium of the corpus callosum. Here it is joined by the **internal cerebral vein**, which emerges from the roof of the third ventricle, under cover of the splenium of the corpus callosum, having drained the choroid plexuses. The basal and internal cerebral veins of the two sides join to form the single **great cerebral vein** (of Galen) which after a short course runs back into the straight sinus.

Select Bibliography

No references are given here to the very large number of articles in learned journals which have been consulted in the preparation of this text. The following is a brief list of books, monographs, and published symposia which have been drawn upon; most of the pertinent references will be found in them.

BAILEY P. & VON BONIN G. *The Isocortex of Man.* University of Illinois Press, Urbana, Ill., 1951.

BONICA J.J. (ed.) *Advances in Neurology. Vol. IV: Pain.* Raven Press, New York, 1974

BOURNE, G.H. (ed.) *Structure and Function of Nervous Tissue.* Academic Press, New York, Vol. I. 1968. Vol. II. 1969.

BOWSHER, D. *Cerebrospinal Fluid Dynamics in Health and Disease.* Charles C. Thomas, Springfield, Ill., 1960.

BRODAL, A., *Neurological Anatomy in Relation to Clinical Medicine,* 2nd edition, Oxford U.P., 1969.

ECCLES, J.C., ITO M. & SZENTHAGOTHAI J. *The Cerebellum as a Neuronal Machine,* Springer, Berlin, 1967.

FIELD, J.H., MAGOUN W. & HALL V.E. (eds.) *Handbook of Physiology: Sections I, II and III: Neurophysiology.* American Physiological Society, Washington, D.C., 1959–61.

FRIGYESI T., RINVIK E. & YAHR M.D. (eds.) *Corticothalamic Projections and Sensorimotor Activities.* Raven Press, New York, 1973.

HODGKIN A.L., *The Conduction of the Nervous Impulse.* Liverpool U.P. 1964.

HUBBARD J.L., LLINAS R. & QUASTEL, D.M.J. *Electrophysiological Analysis of Synaptic Transmission* (Monographs of the Physiological Society, no 19). Edward Arnold, London, 1969.

IGGO A. (ed.) *Handbook of Sensory Physiology. Vol. II: Somatosensory System.* Springer, Berlin, 1973.

JASPER H.H., PROCTOR L.D., KNIGHTON R.S., NOSHAY W.C. & COSTELLO R. (eds.) *Reticular Formation of the Brain* (Henry Ford Hospital International Symposium). Churchill, London, 1958.

LOEWENSTEIN W.R. (ed.) *Handbook of Sensory Physiology. Vol. I: Principles of Receptor Physiology.* Springer, Berlin, 1971.

MATTHEWS P.B.C. *Mammalian Muscle Receptors and their Central Actions* (Monographs of the Physiological Society, no 23). Edward Arnold, London 1972

MELZACK R. *The Puzzle of Pain.* Penguin Books, London, 1973.

MOUNTCASTLE V.B. (ed.) *Medical Physiology.* 12th edition, Vol. II. C.V. Mosby Co., St. Louis, 1968.

SCHMITT, F.O. (ed.) *The Neurosciences: A Study Program.* Rockefeller U.P., New York, 1967.

SCHMITT, F.O. (ed.) *The Neurosciences: Second Study Program.* Rockefeller U.P., New York, 1971.

SCHMITT F.O. & WORDEN F.G. (eds.) *The Neurosciences: Third Study Program.* MIT Press, Cambridge, Mass., 1974.

Index